Health and Healing

Books by Andrew Weil, M.D.

The Natural Mind:
A New Way of Looking at Drugs
and the Higher Consciousness

The Marriage of the Sun and Moon:
A Quest for Unity in Consciousness

Chocolate to Morphine:
Understanding Mind-Active Drugs
(with Winifred Rosen)

Health and Healing:
Understanding Conventional
and Alternative Medicine

Health and Healing
*Understanding Conventional
and Alternative Medicine*

Andrew Weil, M.D.

Houghton Mifflin Company
Boston

Library of Congress Cataloging in Publication Data

Weil, Andrew.
Health and Healing.

Includes index.
1. Therapeutic systems. 2. Medicine. 3. Health.
I. Title.
R733.W44   1983   615.5′3   83-10845
ISBN 0-395-34430-1
ISBN 0-395-37764-1 (pbk.)

Printed in the United States of America

D   9   8   7   6   5

Houghton Mifflin Company paperback, 1985

Acknowledgments

MUCH OF THE MATERIAL in this book grew out of lectures given over the past several years in the Human Behavior and Development course at the College of Medicine of the University of Arizona in Tucson. I am grateful to the creators of that course, Dr. Shirley Nickols Fahey and Dr. Herbert Pollock, for giving me the incentive to organize my information about alternative treatment and my speculations on the importance of placebo responses.

Persons who helped me find facts and references I needed include Dana Ullman, Harris Coulter, Leif Zerkin, Dr. Fred Edwards, Dr. Gregory Manteuffel, Dr. Joseph Alpert, Dr. Guido Majno, and Dr. Bernard Beitman.

Other people helped me by reading portions of the manuscript in its preliminary stages: Winifred Rosen, Willard Johnson, Steve Goehring, Woody Wickham, Sue Fleishman, Dr. Joseph Subasic.

Russell and Hope Williams gave me a place to write when I moved to California in the middle of working on the book. Kim Cliffton kept my energy and spirits up. Zig Schmitt helped me get settled on the East Coast when I left California.

Finally, I would like to thank Anita McClellan and Austin Olney of Houghton Mifflin and Lynn Nesbit of International Creative Management. Their steady interest in the book kept my own from flagging.

CONTENTS

I

TREATMENT AND CURE: THE STRANGE CASE OF HOMEOPATHY

1

A Homeopathic Cure?

IN FEBRUARY OF 1980, while on a business trip to Berkeley, California, I had a sudden attack of a pain I had never before experienced. It started in the center of my chest and eventually radiated to the center of my back, left shoulder, throat, and right lower jaw. The pain was steady, with a penetrating, boring quality. It was associated with a feeling of difficulty in swallowing, as if something were lodged in the very bottom of my esophagus. There were no other symptoms.

The first episode came out of the blue in the evening, two hours after eating a regular meal, when I was relaxing after a stressful day. The pain was unrelieved by drinking water, eating, or doing anything else simple I could think of. It lasted two hours, then subsided as I lay down to sleep. The next morning, it was gone.

My anxiety about this experience was as great as the actual discomfort. I was then thirty-seven and in good health, but as a nonbeliever in regular physical examinations, had not had a general medical checkup in four years. Moreover, my training and background as a physician have made me reluctant to go to doctors or hospitals except for real emergencies. I have practiced paying attention to my body, diagnosing my own problems, and treating them myself whenever I can. As a result of this practice, I have become a sharp observer of changes in my body, usually detecting illnesses at very early stages and having a good sense of their nature.

In this case my intuition gave me some hunches but left a lot of questions. I was quite sure the pain came from my digestive system, probably from the upper end of it. If I'd had to guess,

I would have said it arose from the upper part of the stomach or near the junction of the esophagus and stomach. It had some of the quality of the heartburn I'd had years before in college and medical school when I ate poorly and was much less caring of my body, but it was stronger and seemed to me to indicate a potentially serious problem. The main question was, would it recur?

It did, about a week later, when I was in New York City, again on business and again during a stressful time. The second episode started in the morning, just after eating a light breakfast. It got so bad, I had to lie down and give up trying to work on an article I wanted to finish writing. This time I tried taking an antacid — baking soda was the only one available in the apartment I was staying in. It helped for a few minutes, but the pain quickly returned, more persistent and penetrating than ever. It lasted most of the morning, finally disappearing around noon. Eating lunch did not reactivate it.

In the next week, it recurred three times, generally lasting longer and making me steadily more anxious. Now there was no doubt that something was wrong.

For many men of my age and their doctors, pain in the chest can be especially alarming as a symptom of heart disease. My intuitive sense that the pain came from my digestive tract was strong enough to allay any fears I had about my heart. To be absolutely sure, I went for a run during one occurrence of the pain and satisfied myself that it had no correlation with exertion. My heart and lungs behaved normally. I could also find no correlation with time of day or with intake of any particular kind or quantity of food or drink. Nor could I find an effective method to get relief.

After these distressing recurrences, I returned home to Arizona, and the symptom went away. For two weeks I had not a twinge of it. Then, suddenly, it started up again, once waking me up from sleep at night, once lasting all day, and once starting within minutes of finishing a carbonated drink and reaching a new level of intensity.

Running over all the possibilities I could think of, I came up with five, none of them cheering. The first and strongest was ulcer, but ulcer pain should be relieved by eating and antacids; this was not. Also, intuition tells me I am not an ulcer type. The second possibility was hiatal hernia, in which a portion of the stomach protrudes upward through the diaphragm around the esophagus. That condition is usually accompanied by other signs of indigestion and is relieved by lying down with the upper part of the body elevated. I had no other digestive symptoms and got no relief from changes in position. A third possibility was gall bladder disease, but gall bladder pain usually comes regularly after eating, is more common at night, and rarely lasts more than three hours. My pain had no consistent relationship to meals, was long lasting, and was more frequent in daytime.

A fourth possibility was some sort of parasite in the upper intestinal tract. I had made a number of visits to the South American tropics and had not been tested for parasites in a long time. I liked this possibility best, because it would be an external cause, easily treated. I knew the location of the pain and absence of intestinal symptoms were against it, but I eagerly submitted stool samples to a laboratory for examination. They were consistently negative for parasites. Finally, a pancreatic problem was a possibility, although an exceedingly slim one, and, again, intuition told me that was not it.

I still was not ready to go to a doctor, because I did not (or did not want to) consider the problem a real emergency. Instead, I talked it over with a friend who was finishing a medical internship at the University of Arizona Health Sciences Center. I had met him when I lectured to his freshman medical school class and had become friends with him over his student years. I trusted his book knowledge of orthodox medicine, since it was much fresher than mine.

My friend felt that ulcer was the most likely answer, that I should try aggressive treatment with strong antacids and submit to diagnostic X-rays if the pain continued. It did continue, and strong antacids did not affect it. Reluctantly, I decided to consult a gastroenterologist. Six weeks had passed since the first occurrence. The episodes were now more frequent and more severe. I could find no remedy, and I had no clear understanding of what was wrong. I try to act as my own physician, as I have said, but in so doing I stay very aware of the limits of my knowledge and experience. This problem was out of the range of my previous experience and lay beyond those limits.

My intern friend recommended a gastroenterologist he liked

both professionally and personally. I made an appointment for a few days hence and resigned myself to being a patient.

On the day I went to his hospital office I had no pain. I recited my story to the doctor, precisely describing the symptom and my sense of it. He listened, examined me briefly, then told me his opinion. He said I had given him almost a textbook description of the pain of esophageal spasm: an episodic constriction of the muscular tube that carries food to the stomach. The spasm occurs near the junction with the stomach and is often of unknown cause. It is not usually associated with any more serious pathology of the gastrointestinal tract and can be alleviated, if not eliminated, by adjusting diet, experimenting with antacids and changes in position, and other methods. The gastroenterologist sent me to have an electrocardiogram to make sure I had no heart problem (I didn't), then wrote out a requisition to the X-ray department for a barium swallow, in order to prove the diagnosis of esophageal spasm.

Drinking a preparation of barium sulfate makes the esophagus visible on X-ray. I would have to wait until I was having the pain to take this test; only then would any constriction in the esophagus be apparent. If it did not show up, it might be brought out by adding some hydrochloric acid to the barium to simulate irritation from stomach acid. An instruction for this procedure was included in the X-ray requisition.

I left the hospital in better spirits than I had been in for weeks. My condition had a name. It was not nearly as serious as ulcer or most of the other possibilities I had considered. I did not have to go through extensive diagnostic tests, and the treatments did not sound horrible. Best of all, my intuition was confirmed: the pain originated just where I thought it did. I had no doubt the barium swallow would confirm the presumptive diagnosis of esophageal spasm.

I rather hoped the pain would return that day or the next in order to get confirmation by X-ray, because I had to leave for San Francisco the following day for a week of business. It did not so oblige me, however, and I was unable to do the barium swallow before I left.

On the way to San Francisco, I had a sudden inspiration. I had been meaning to look up another doctor friend, a young man who, after a number of years of working as an emergency room physician, had become a homeopath. He now practiced at a homeopathic clinic in Berkeley and also saw private patients in Marin County. He had been wanting me to visit so he could tell me about his new career.

I had long been interested in homeopathy, but my knowledge of it came mainly from reading. I had never consulted a homeopathic practitioner nor watched one at work. In learning about different systems of medicine, I have found it essential to seek experience of them as well as intellectual knowledge. The best way I know to do that is to present myself as a patient and see what happens. A limitation to this method is that it requires some need for treatment. If I am generally healthy, as I usually am, I cannot play the role of patient satisfactorily.

Now I had a real symptom, one that cried out for relief. This would be a perfect opportunity to be a homeopathic patient and see what that system could do for me. Since the gastroenterologist in Tucson did not seem to have any sure-fire cures to offer, I had all the more reason to seek a remedy elsewhere.

My friend, Dr. Greg Manteuffel, told me how his dissatisfaction with conventional medicine led him to explore other forms of treatment and finally apprentice himself to a homeopath in Chicago. In this course, he followed in the path of most of the homeopaths in history; most have been M.D.'s who rejected the methods they first learned, then studied the theory and practice of homeopathy as apprentices to established practitioners of that system.

My friend told me he was much more successful in treating people since his conversion; he was also much happier, had better rapport with patients, and for the first time in his life really enjoyed practicing medicine. He felt he was able to stimulate genuine healing in sick people, whereas before he just suppressed symptoms, often by plying patients with toxic drugs and using other methods he now considered more harmful than beneficial.

I proposed that he show me how he practiced by taking me on as a new patient, especially since I had a recent health problem that had been bothering me. He agreed, going right to work by doing an "intake" on me, which is the homeopathic equivalent of a medical history. Sitting across from me with a notepad, he began to ask me questions.

The questions went on for a very long time. Many of them seemed strange, certainly not the kinds of questions I was taught to ask patients as an allopathic* doctor. For example: Are you a warm person or a cold person? What position do you sleep in? Do you like the fat part of meat or the lean? Do you feel better under clear skies or cloudy? Do you crave any flavors of food?

There were familiar questions about symptoms also, but Greg wanted to know all my symptoms, even the ones that seemed trivial to me, and he did not seem to attach greater importance to those I thought were the big ones, like my pain. He wanted to know all about the pain, but only from my subjective point of view: its quality, duration, location, and so forth. He could not have cared less about the name "esophageal spasm" so recently attached to it, nor about my speculations on its nature. He recorded the pain as just one entry in a comprehensive list of all my complaints, regarding it as only one detail of a larger picture. I would never have thought to mention most of the other symptoms to the gastroenterologist; to my mind (and surely to his) they would have been irrelevant to the story of the pain in my digestive tract. They included a tendency to neck stiffness, a sore left knee, depression, occasional skin eruptions, sore throats from time to time, and so forth.

At the end of the questioning, which took more than an hour, Greg made a number of notes on his pad, then looked up and gave me his diagnosis as a homeopath. He told me I had given him almost a textbook description of the symptoms provoked by elemental sulfur.

Homeopaths believe people get sick in individual ways, showing distinctive patterns of symptoms. Whether one person's symptoms resemble another person's symptoms is of no import. Homeopaths do not believe in the existence of "disease entities" like hepatitis or ulcer common to many patients with similar

---

*The usual kind of medicine practiced by M.D.'s is called "allopathic" to distinguish it from homeopathic and other therapeutic systems. The origin of that term is explained in the next chapter (p. 17). I use "allopathic medicine" interchangeably with "regular medicine," "orthodox medicine," "conventional medicine," and "scientific medicine."

symptoms. Rather, they concern themselves only with identifying the particular pattern of symptoms of an individual patient, and this they do by means of the curious questioning I went through. Little emphasis is placed on physical diagnosis — on examination or testing of the patient.

Once the symptom pattern is clear, the homeopath then tries to match it with the one substance that most closely reproduces these symptoms in the normal person. The method here is to consult large volumes of "provings" that homeopaths have compiled over the years. These are records in great detail of the results of giving small amounts of many different substances to volunteer subjects in good health. Simple chemicals, minerals, extracts of plants, dilute preparations of animal and insect venoms and of disease-causing germs, as well as of some standard drugs, are all included in the homeopathic provings. It is most important to match the patient's symptoms with the one substance that most closely reproduces them, because homeopathy asserts that a single dose of that substance, highly diluted and properly prepared, has the capacity to cure the ailing patient.

In my case the match was easily made, because elemental sulfur is a common and familiar homeopathic remedy that rapidly produces very clear symptoms. Apparently I was a recognizable sulfur type. Greg invited me to meet him in Berkeley the next day at the clinic where he worked. He wanted me to watch him process patients there and promised to give me his homeopathic prescription — a single, tiny dose of sulfur that he felt would give me good results.

The Hering Family Health Clinic looked like a clinic, complete with nurses and visiting medical students, but it lacked much of the paraphernalia of an allopathic facility. There was a pharmacy and a library filled with the works of the chief theorists of homeopathy, along with many editions of the homeopathic materia medica and provings.

I sat with Greg as he talked with several patients, doing intakes on new ones, reviewing the charts and checking on the progress of old ones. The patients were a cross section of Berkeley's heterogeneous population, no different from those I would expect to find as outpatients in a regular hospital in that city. One middle-aged Englishwoman told me how delighted she had been to discover the clinic. She had used homeopathic doctors all her life and had feared that on moving to California she would not be able to find one.

At the end of the morning, Greg gave me a small vial partly filled with tiny white pellets. The pellets, he told me, were lactose — milk sugar — on which he had placed a drop of a dilute suspension of sulfur. One of the most peculiar tenets of homeopathy, and the one that makes it least comprehensible to orthodox scientists and doctors, is that substances become more powerful as remedies when they are diluted. Some homeopathic remedies are such extreme dilutions that little or none of the original substance is present. Yet these "high potencies," as they are called, are the very preparations said to be most powerful and requiring most caution to prescribe. What possible sense can a conventional doctor make of that belief?

The dose of sulfur I got was a fairly high dilution. Greg told me to place the contents of the vial on my tongue, let it dissolve, then drink some water. He also told me that sulfur is one of the quicker-acting remedies and that he was sure it was the right treatment for me. He cautioned me to avoid from then on all coffee and any form of camphor, for either external or internal use. These two substances are homeopathic antidotes that will negate the therapeutic effect of a remedy even years later. (Not being a coffee drinker, I would not find this advice difficult to follow.) I thanked Greg and left the clinic, not quite sure how I felt about this method of diagnosis and treatment. Reading about it was one thing. Experiencing it as a patient was another.

The rest of this story is quickly told. I never was able to have my barium swallow, because the pain never returned, not once in the two years that have passed since the time of my visits to a gastroenterologist and a homeopath. I have had no digestive or other serious problems and continue to avoid coffee and camphor.

I begin with this bit of personal history because it includes all the themes I wish to discuss in this book. What is health? What is illness? What is healing? What is treatment and what is its relationship to cure? How can you take personal responsibility for health, and when do you need to seek outside help? What kind of outside help should you seek?

The medical experience I have recounted here has a happy

outcome. I am cured. Perhaps as a patient I should let it go at that and not wonder what happened. As a doctor and investigator, I cannot. I have a terrible curiosity to know what was wrong with me and why it went away. Actually, I have that curiosity as a patient, too, because when I need help with a medical problem next time, I want to know what I should do.

Perhaps I should do nothing. One possibility is that the problem, whatever it was, ran its course and disappeared. Very many problems do that if left alone, providing a good rationale for conservative management of illness. If there is not a fulminating emergency, it rarely hurts to do nothing but watch. Of course, in this case, I had done nothing for six weeks, and my pain was becoming more and more familiar. Nothing in its course suggested that it was about to make a sudden farewell.

Another possibility is to go to a conventional doctor and get a name for the problem. "Esophageal spasm" was music to my ears. It turned the pain into a concrete, known, and not very grave condition, instantly reducing my anxiety. Until then, my imagination had busily fed nightmarish possibilities into my consciousness, which certainly could not have helped my digestive system. If my pain had some relation to stress — a reasonable assumption, since the stomach and esophagus are very responsive to changes in mental and emotional state — then the reduction of stress caused by finding a name for the problem might have permitted it to subside and heal naturally, whatever it was. Naming diseases is one of the bugaboos of homeopathy, but it can provide tremendous reassurance to worried patients with active imaginations (assuming, of course that the name is not "cancer" or something equally frightening).

As for homeopathy, what about its role in this saga? Was I cured by that dose of homeopathic sulfur? It certainly looks that way, and the experience was impressive enough to persuade me to go to a homeopath again next time I need outside help for a medical problem. Still, my restless mind will not let me be comfortable with that conclusion. If homeopathy cured me, I must know how it did so.

2

Like Cures Like, and Less Is More

HOMEOPATHY DATES FORMALLY from 1810, the year of publication of Samuel Christian Hahnemann's most important work, the *Organon of Medicine*. Hahnemann was a German physician who lived from 1755 to 1843. As recently as a century ago, he was considered one of the greatest heroes of modern medicine. Hospitals all over the world still carry his name, and a statue of him in Washington, D.C., bears only the inscription HAHNEMANN, without other identification of any kind. Yet few doctors or medical students today could tell you who he was or why he became so famous.[1]

As a child, Hahnemann displayed a prodigious intellect, with special facility for learning languages. He studied medicine at good academic centers, including universities in Leipzig and Vienna, receiving his M.D. in 1779. After graduation, he became an itinerant physician but soon lost faith in the methods he had learned. He could not get good results from them and came to consider them dangerous, especially the administration of drugs he felt were not understood. Instead he recommended exercise, good diet, and fresh air to the patients he treated. Hahnemann was not a success as a traditional doctor. Finally, he gave up his practice altogether, resolving to make a living as a translator.

To understand Hahnemann's dissatisfaction, it is necessary to know what orthodox medicine was like in his day. The period from about 1780 to 1850 was known as the Age of Heroic Medicine because of the reckless vigor of its methods. The favorite heroic treatment was bleeding. Bleeding was accomplished in various ways, the commonest and most effective being venesection — that is, the slitting of a vein with a lancet or sharp blade.

It was usual to let a pint of blood at a time, sometimes more, and to repeat the process at frequent intervals. (The prestigious British medical journal *The Lancet* traces its history to the days of heroic practice; hence the name.)

Orthodox medicine in the late 1700s was an exclusively male, elitist enterprise, taught in universities closed to women. The University of Edinburgh had the leading medical school of the period, and its professor of physic, William Cullen, was the chief theoretician of heroic practice. Cullen believed in a unitary theory of disease. He felt that all symptoms resulted from one underlying cause: bad blood. The remedy was to remove it.

Cullen's chief disciple in America was Benjamin Rush, a signer of the Declaration of Independence and heroic physician par excellence. Rush carried bleeding to an extreme. He bled one patient eighty-five times in six months, removed eight pints of blood from another over six weeks, and is credited with saying: "I would rather die with my Lancet in my hand than give it up while I had Breath to maintain it or a hand to use it."[2]

Bleeding was supplemented by several other treatments designed to remove impurities and toxins from the body. Intestinal purging was held in high esteem, and the drug most often used to produce it was calomel (mercurous chloride). Heroic doctors gave their patients huge doses of calomel, following the current teaching to administer it until the patient began to salivate freely, a sign that the drug was working. Toxicology texts today list salivation as an early sign of acute mercury intoxication, one of the most dangerous forms of heavy metal poisoning.

In addition to purging, vomiting was induced by giving violent emetic drugs such as tartar emetic, a poisonous antimony salt. Other drugs, called diaphoretics, were used to cause profuse sweating. Blistering was carried out by rubbing or burning local irritants on the skin, including cantharides (Spanish fly). In "cupping," a heated glass cup was placed on the skin; as it cooled, a partial vacuum drew blood to the site, which was then lanced as another way of drawing off the bad fluid.

In the light of today's knowledge, it is certain that heroic medicine sped many patients on to their final rest. Here is an account of the death of George Washington:

Even George Washington, who received the best medical care of the day, spent his last hours undergoing heroic treatment. On December 14, 1799, the former President came down with a severe sore throat. It was inflamed and gave him some difficulty in breathing. His overseer removed a pint of blood, but it provided no relief. A physician was called, who soon after his arrival applied a blister to the throat and let another pint of blood. At three o'clock in the afternoon, two other doctors came to consult with the first one, and by a vote of two to one, they decided to let more blood, removing a quart at that time. They reported that the blood flowed "slow and thick." By then the President was dehydrated, and it would seem that the doctors must have had to squeeze out the final drops of blood. Washington died sometime between ten and eleven that same night. In his case heroic treatment consisted of the removal of at least four pints of blood, blistering, and a dose of calomel. Perhaps he would have died in any case, but the treatment certainly provided no relief.[3]

A few physicians of the time opposed these heroic measures, but they were a distinct minority. Other traditions of healing existed as well. For example, country women in Europe and America practiced herbalism, sometimes with great success and at least without causing much direct harm. No university-trained male physician would have anything to do with them.

Samuel Hahnemann rejected heroic medicine after giving it a brief try because it ran counter to his intuitive convictions about health and healing. A deeply religious man, steeped in the mysticism of Emanuel Swedenborg, Hahnemann believed that healing came from God and Nature and needed only to be gently encouraged by the physician. He was especially disturbed by what he considered the thoughtless prescription of toxic drugs.

Beginning his new career as a translator, Hahnemann set out in 1790 to prepare a German edition of William Cullen's *Materia Medica*. As the work proceeded, his conviction grew that Cullen's prescriptions lacked an experimental basis. How could you give drugs to sick people if you did not understand their actions on normal people? Only experimental determination of the effects of drugs would allow a physician to prescribe them wisely.

Accordingly, Hahnemann drew up a set of rules for testing drugs. Though he is never given credit for it, he is really the father of experimental pharmacology, and pharmacologists today might still benefit from reading his suggestions. Here are some of the rules as they eventually appeared in the *Organon of Medicine*:[4]

— Therefore medicines on which depend man's life and death, disease and health, must be thoroughly and most carefully distinguished from one another, and for this purpose tested by careful pure experiments on the healthy body for the purpose of ascertaining their powers and real effects . . .

— Each of these medicines must be taken in a perfectly simple, unadulterated form; the indigenous plants in the form of freshly expressed juice, mixed with a little alcohol to prevent it spoiling; exotic vegetable substances, however, in the form of powder, or tincture prepared with alcohol when they were in the fresh state, and afterward mingled with a certain proportion of water; salts and gums, however, should be dissolved in water just before being taken.

— For these experiments every medicinal substance must be employed quite alone and perfectly pure, without the admixture of any foreign substance, and without taking anything else of a medicinal nature on the same day, nor yet on the subsequent days, nor during all the time we wish to observe the effects of the medicine.

— During all the time the experiment lasts, the diet must be strictly regulated; it should be as much as possible destitute of spices, of a purely nutritious and simple character . . . The drinks are to be those usually partaken of, as little stimulating as possible.

— The medicines must be tested on both males and females, in order also to reveal the alterations of health they produce in the sexual sphere.

— If the effects that result from such a dose [i.e., an initial dilution] are but slight, a few more globules may be taken daily, until they become more distinct and stronger and the alterations of the health are more conspicuous; for all persons are not affected by a medicine in an equally great degree; on the contrary, there is a vast variety in this respect . . .

— The best provings of the pure effects of simple medicines in altering the human health, and of the artificial diseases and symptoms they are capable of developing in the healthy individual are those which the healthy, unprejudiced, and sensitive *physician institutes on himself* with all the caution and care here enjoined. He knows with the greatest certainty the things he has experienced in his own person.

I reproduce these passages from the *Organon* both to give the flavor of Hahnemann's writing and also to point out some of his wisdom. These suggestions strike me as very sensible, all the more so because modern drug testing consistently violates them. For example, Hahnemann's admonition to test drugs equally on men and women is ignored today; governmental regulations virtually exclude women as subjects in drug research. As a result, we do not know how the drugs we use might affect the sexes differently. His point about a "vast variety" in ways people respond to the same medicine is also important. Medical students today learn effects of drugs as if they were automatic and invariable. As young doctors, they are often quite surprised to find that actual patients do not respond as pharmacology texts and pharmaceutical advertising say they should.

Of course, the idea of self-experimentation by physicians has gone completely out the window. In fact, the doctor today who tries out drugs on himself is likely to be accused of unprofessional conduct. Hahnemann's followers not only thought it unethical to give others drugs they had not first self-tested, they also believed that was the best method to understand a drug's effects.

In this spirit, Hahnemann set out to "prove" on himself the common remedies of his day, following the careful rules he had devised. The first experiment he made was with cinchona bark, and it led him to formulate the first of three laws that became the basis of a new system of medicine.

Cinchona, also known as Peruvian bark or Jesuits' bark, comes from a tropical South American tree of the coffee family. It is the natural source of quinine and was used by South American Indians to treat fevers, especially those of malaria. Spanish physicians and Jesuit priests began using cinchona in Lima in the mid-1600s, and their successes with it led to a great demand for the bark in Europe, where malaria was also prevalent. Not only was cinchona the first effective treatment for malaria, it was also the first *specific* to enter Western medicine: a particular remedy for a particular disease.

William Cullen thought that cinchona worked by strengthening the stomach because it was bitter and astringent — a guess with no basis in experimental observation. To test it, Hahnemann compounded a remedy that was more bitter and more astringent than cinchona and showed it to be useless in treating the relapsing fevers of malaria. Next, while in good health, he took a dose of the bark himself and found it made him feverish.[5] This experience, later reinforced by many experiments with many substances, gave him the first part of his new theory, which he called the Law of Similars. Put simply, it states, "Like cures like." A slightly expanded version is: "A substance that produces a certain set of symptoms in a healthy person has the power to cure a sick person manifesting those same symptoms." Hahnemann coined a new word, *homeopathy*, to describe medical treatment based on the Law of Similars, putting it together from Greek roots meaning "like the disease."

The opposite of treatment by similars is treatment by contraries, and Hahnemann called this practice antipathy. Giving aspirin to lower fever or prescribing antihypertensive drugs to treat high blood pressure are examples of antipathic medicine. Hahnemann coined another word to describe the regular, heroic medicine his contemporaries practiced. He called it allopathic, from Greek roots meaning "other than the disease," because he felt it prescribed drugs on the basis of no consistent or logical relationship to symptoms. The name has stuck to this day, though few allopathic physicians know its origin or meaning.

As Hahnemann continued his provings of drugs and began to treat patients by the Law of Similars, he observed a biphasic pattern in drug effects. Often an initial set of symptoms would be followed some time later by an opposite set. Opium, for example, produces euphoria and stimulation at the outset but depression later on. Hahnemann interpreted this pattern as one of action and reaction, the initial symptoms being direct drug effects, the delayed ones the body's attempt to restore equilibrium.

Perhaps homeopathic treatment worked by mobilizing the body to react against the disease, especially since administering a similar drug often produced an immediate worsening of symptoms, followed by cure. In an effort to moderate the initial effect, Hahnemann tried reducing the dosages of his remedies. To his surprise, they became more powerful. His religious beliefs led him to consider spiritual reality more important than material reality; applying this attitude to therapeutics, he came to regard the spiritual essence of a drug as more important than its physical substance. His philosophy, combined with the results of his experiments, brought Hahnemann to the second law of homeopathy, known as the Law of Infinitesimals. It states (to the eternal dismay of allopaths) that the smaller the dose of a remedy, when properly diluted, the more effective it will be at stimulating the body's vital forces to react against disease.

Hahnemann worked out a precise method for diluting remedies to maximize their effectiveness. Beginning with the original substance — say the fresh juice of a medicinal plant preserved with a little alcohol — he would put one part of it in nine parts of an 87 percent solution of alcohol and distilled water. He then "succussed" the vial of solution by forcibly striking it one hundred times against a leather pad. Hahnemann does not state how he hit upon this technique or discovered its ability to intensify the power of a remedy. He believed that succussion "dynamized," or activated, the therapeutic potential of a drug. He wrote: "Homeopathic dynamizations are processes by which the medicinal properties of drugs, which are in a latent state in the crude substance, are excited and enabled to act spiritually (dynamically) upon the vital forces."[6]

The result of the first step in this process is a one-in-ten dilution, called the 1X dilution in homeopathic shorthand. One part of this in nine parts of diluent, succussed 100 times, makes the 2X dilution, and so on up to 30X, 200X, and beyond. The early preparations are called "low" dilutions, the later ones "high" or "extreme." By the Law of Infinitesimals, each succeeding dilution will be more powerful than the last.

Hahnemann proposed a rule for treatment with these diluted drugs: the single-remedy rule. It enjoins the physician to use only one homeopathic remedy at a time, waiting to see what happens before taking further action, never to use two or more simultaneously.

With the two laws of homeopathy, the rule of the single remedy, and a growing list of provings of drugs, Hahnemann embarked on a career as a new kind of physician. After nearly twenty years of practice, he added one last law to the theoretical framework of his system. He called it the Law of Chronic Disease and used it to explain why treatment based on the first two laws did not always work. He found many cases in which homeopathic treatment produced relief of acute symptoms, only to have the symptoms recur at a later date or be replaced by a new pattern of complaints.

The Law of Chronic Disease states that when disease persists despite treatment it is the result of one or more conditions that affect many people and have been driven deep inside the body by earlier allopathic therapy. The law named three such conditions (Hahnemann called them "miasms"): psora ("the itch"), syphilis, and sycosis (or gonorrhea). Hahnemann used the term *psora* to cover a whole range of itching, inflamed states of the skin. As long as they remained on the body surface, they caused nothing worse than discomfort, but if allopathic medicine suppressed the symptoms of this condition, driving it inside the body, it could reappear years later in the form of diseases as diverse as diabetes, cancer, arthritis, and schizophrenia. Before a homeopath could treat such problems, he would first have to treat the underlying chronic disease.*

The Law of Chronic Disease was the weakest of Hahnemann's theories, causing much argument among his followers. Homeopaths today still recognize and treat three patterns of chronic disease but no longer think they are causally connected to specific acute infections like gonorrhea and syphilis. They also still wrestle with the problem of why homeopathic treatment does not always work.

As we shall see in the course of this book, no system of treat-

---

*The Law of Chronic Disease sounds archaic, but it contains an idea worth studying: namely, that disease on the surface of the body is less serious than disease in the interior. Homeopaths believe that the appearance of skin eruptions following treatment of internal disease is a hopeful sign of healing, and they regard suppression of superficial symptoms as a great mistake. I know of no research to support or discredit those beliefs, but since they are empirical findings of homeopaths, I am willing to consider them.

The immune system is an important key to many unexplained diseases and cures. Allergic skin reactions such as hives, eczema, and other forms of dermatitis are not uncommon in the histories of patients who develop more serious diseases, such as rheumatoid arthritis, systemic lupus erythematosus, and multiple sclerosis, which may also represent unbalanced immunological functioning. Allopathic medicine has come up with much more effective ways of suppressing itching, inflamed states of the skin than it had in Hahnemann's day. The corticosteroids — synthetic drugs related to the adrenal hormone cortisone — powerfully prevent expression of such reactions but may not correct the underlying cause. Steroid therapy often makes dermatological problems recede in the short run, but what are its long-term consequences for the immune system? The homeopathic experience makes me wonder.

ment works all the time. Every system, however scientific, clever, and refined, fails some of the time, and it is interesting to see how its practitioners interpret the failures. Hahnemann tried to blame some of his on meddling by his rivals, the allopaths.

In general, homeopathy's successes far outshone its failures in the years after Hahnemann first presented the new system to the world. By ones and twos, then by dozens, then by hundreds, physicians in Europe gave up the practice of allopathy to follow Hahnemann's teachings. They and their patients were delighted by the results, and their accumulated experience made it possible to refine and perfect the art of homeopathic therapeutics. When Hahnemann died in 1843 at the age of eighty-eight, he was successful and wealthy, and the medical heresy he had launched seemed destined to establish itself throughout the Western world.[7]

The seeds of homeopathy fell on particularly fertile soil in America. The first homeopathic physician arrived in the United States in 1828. Eight years later, the Hahnemann Medical College opened in Philadelphia. Hahnemann's works were available in English by the early 1840s. An American Institute of Homeopathy, founded in 1844, became the first national medical society. Most significant, American homeopaths did much better than allopaths in treating victims of cholera epidemics that swept through the Midwest at the end of the 1840s. Their success brought them prestige and money and encouraged widespread desertions from the ranks of orthodox practitioners. By 1850 another homeopathic medical college had opened in Cleveland.

Throughout this period, American medicine was in great political turmoil. As far back as 1772, well before Hahnemann had his M.D., regular doctors in the American colonies began to organize and secure legislation favorable to themselves. Soon after independence, they set up state medical societies and mechanisms for licensing physicians, always with the intent to exclude from practice "irregular" doctors who were not schooled and approved by the orthodox establishment. In 1807 a law went on the books in New York State setting a five-dollar fine for each month of practice by an unlicensed doctor. An 1827 law gave only licensed practitioners the right to use the New York courts to recover unpaid fees.

The excesses of heroic medicine and the arrogant political behavior of its practitioners produced a strong reaction among the citizens of the young country. Jacksonian democrats, who viewed all monopolies as the enemies of freedom, opposed the medical licensing laws as antidemocratic. They joined forces with all those who disapproved of heroic medical care to form a powerful political tide known as the Popular Health Movement. The goal of the Popular Health Movement was nothing less than the repeal of all medical licensing laws, allowing people who considered themselves qualified to practice any form of healing they deemed worthwhile. The movement was very effective in achieving its goals. It gained control of one state legislature after another and by the end of the 1840s had wiped nearly all of the licensing laws off the books. Regular doctors were routed.

Conventional histories of medicine portray the Popular Health Movement as the darkest period of American medicine. In many ways it does not seem so. It was a time of great experimentation in matters of health. There was a trend toward self-responsibility, summed up in the slogan "Every man his own doctor." A strong women's movement coexisted with the Popular Health Movement, emphasizing preventive care and providing courses for women to learn about their own bodies. Resentment of regular doctors ran high, and with justification. Not only did they bleed and purge people to death, they tried to put out of business competitors who attempted to heal the sick with gentler methods.[8]

Into this turbulent atmosphere came homeopathy. Its disciples were meticulous observers of the most basic injunction on doctors: *primum non nocere* — first, do no harm.* With their minute doses of remedies, they could not possibly make patients worse. Early homeopaths were aglow with the zeal of new converts. They had a comprehensive theory of health, disease, and treatment, based in experimental research and handed down by a master. They were concerned with patients as individuals. They aimed to cure disease from within, at its source, not just suppress symptoms. Best of all, their method worked, even for the gravest infectious illnesses. The Popular Health Movement succeeded just in time to give homeopathy a firm foothold in the New World.

What followed, predictably, was a desperate struggle by the

*Attributed to Hippocrates.

allopaths to regain their lost prestige and control. Then ensued a long and bitter war between allopaths and homeopaths that was fought in every city and town, in virtually every hospital across America.

First the allopaths organized, this time into a much more cohesive and effective political lobby, the American Medical Association, formed in 1846. The following year the new association adopted its code of ethics, which contained the famous "consultation clause": "No one can be considered a regular practitioner, or a fit associate in consultation, whose practice is based upon an exclusive dogma, to the rejection of the accumulated experience of the profession." *Exclusive dogma* was a code phrase for homeopathy. The battle lines were drawn.

Champions of regular medicine began to turn out propaganda against Hahnemann's system. One of the earliest attacks was an 1842 pamphlet titled "Homeopathy and Its Kindred Delusions," written by Oliver Wendell Holmes, a professor at Harvard Medical School. Another move of the allopaths was to try to redefine the name Hahnemann had given them.

Look in a dictionary today and you will sometimes find two very different definitions of *allopathy*. The first is Hahnemann's, based on Greek roots. The second is from German roots meaning "all therapies" and identifies allopathy as a system of medicine that embraces all methods of proven value in the treatment of disease. That revisionist definition dates back only to the mid-1800s, when embattled allopaths, unable to shake their new name, tried to give it a better sound.

From the start, the AMA was militant and exclusive. In 1855 it demanded that all state medical societies accept the code of ethics, requiring them to expel any homeopathic members. In the 1860s the AMA began to bring charges against allopaths who were found to have consulted with homeopaths. It also worked to gain control of city hospitals and boards of health, threatening boycotts of hospitals if homeopaths got privileges at them. During the Civil War, it was able to prevent homeopaths from enlisting in the Army Medical Corps.

In 1868 the AMA refused to admit well-qualified women M.D.'s. In 1870 it refused to seat delegates from racially integrated medical societies and also refused admittance to the Massachusetts

Medical Society unless it purged itself of homeopaths. In 1871, on the occasion of the District of Columbia Medical Society's refusal to admit an M.D. who was accused of violating the code of ethics by having served on the same board of health as a homeopath, the *New York Times* wrote in an editorial: "There is no stronger tenet in the orthodox creed than that it is better the patient should die under the old remedies than recover under homeopathic treatment."[9] In 1878 a Connecticut physician was expelled from his county medical society for consulting with his wife, who happened to be a homeopath.

The ruthlessness of organized allopathy was quickly successful. Achievements of the Popular Health Movement were erased, with licensing laws back on the books in all states, and homeopaths were systematically hounded out of positions of power and importance. Several factors accounted for this reversal. In the first place, the political coalition responsible for the Popular Health Movement dissolved. Second, regular doctors began to abandon the heroic practices that had stirred such resentment. For example, in the 1860s they started using narcotics and alcohol in place of bleeding and calomel. That may not sound like a tremendous advance, but it was. Opiates and alcohol do not kill people outright. Third, homeopathy was beset by internal strife that weakened it as a political force.

In response to unrelenting pressure from allopaths, many homeopaths began to change their ways. Some turned to less dilute forms of remedies. Some added other kinds of treatments to their repertory. Some questioned Hahnemann's teachings. Eventually, American homeopathy was torn apart by dissension. In 1880 the profession split into two groups. The minority, adhering strictly to the master's tenets, became known as Hahnemannians. They remained pure homeopaths, committed to extreme dilutions and the single-remedy rule. The majority said they wanted to modernize, to be able to consult with their allopathic colleagues, to be free of the laborious constraints on practice laid down by Hahnemann. Many of them began to use large doses of allopathic medicines along with homeopathic treatment.

By the end of the nineteenth century, these dissidents had mostly turned into allopaths and were absorbed by the AMA, leaving the minority Hahnemannians to carry on the traditions of homeopathy. Still, in 1900 there were more than fifteen thousand homeopathic practitioners in the United States, one sixth of the entire medical profession. There were also twenty-two homeopathic medical colleges.

The surviving homeopaths were more respectable by then as well. Newer medical heresies, such as osteopathy and chiropractic, seemed much more threatening to the AMA, making homeopathy look established and conservative by comparison. (In 1903, New Jersey's homeopaths and allopaths united to oppose a bill in the legislature to allow licensing of osteopaths.) Respectability notwithstanding, the twentieth century was to bring an almost total decline of homeopathy in America. By 1923 only two of the homeopathic schools were still functioning, and their days were numbered.

The rise of scientific medicine with its great triumphs over infectious illness, its successive discoveries of vitamins, life-giving hormones, antibiotics, and other wonder drugs, won patients away from homeopathy, which came to look stodgy and old-fashioned as the new century progressed. Allopathic medical schools were reorganized and strengthened to ensure that doctors received good education in the basic sciences. Throughout the first half of the 1900s, technology seemed the answer to all humanity's problems, including disease. Allopaths embraced it enthusiastically, while homeopathy stayed the same as it was a hundred years previously, unaffected by technological progress. By midcentury, practicing homeopaths in America were few, and those few were old.

In most of Western Europe, too, homeopathy was totally eclipsed by scientific medicine, but in Third World countries it continued to shine. India has been its adopted home in modern times. There are more homeopaths in India than in any other country today, and most of the English translations of Hahnemann's works are available only from Indian publishing houses. Homeopathic pharmacies and practitioners abound in Latin America as well, although how many of them follow Hahnemann's system strictly is not clear. Homeopathy also flourishes in England, France, Greece, some Eastern European countries, and Sri Lanka.

American homeopathy is now having a modest resurgence, but much of it is suspect. Many non-M.D.'s, including naturopaths, chiropractors, and others not trained in the classical method, now practice what they call homeopathy. Often, they give many remedies at once, ignoring Hahnemann's injunction to use no more than one at a time. Homeopathic remedies have even appeared in health food stores as if they were kinds of dietary supplements. Yet some serious M.D.'s, like my friend in Berkeley, have converted to homeopathy in the traditional way, after losing faith in allopathic medicine.

If homeopathy makes a comeback in the Western world, it will happen because attitudes similar to those prevalent during the Popular Health Movement are again on the rise. In the last quarter of this century, the technological dream that supported allopathy has begun to fade. Dissatisfaction with regular medicine grows year by year in every sector of society, with the same three complaints voiced over and over: it has become too expensive, too dangerous, and not effective enough at treating the diseases that really matter, such as heart disease, cancer, and stroke. Modern hospital medicine looks more and more "heroic" in its reliance on invasive procedures that depend on elaborate technology and seem to ignore or deny the body's own healing powers.

If allopathic enmity toward homeopathy has subsided, it is only because homeopathy no longer poses an economic threat to regular practitioners. Intellectually, it is as threatening as ever, since its philosophy is totally at odds with that of scientific medicine. Allopathy is rooted in materialism. Homeopathy, in both theory and practice, attaches greater importance to nonmaterial reality. For the allopathic theorist, the continued existence of homeopathy must be galling. That homeopathy works is even more of an affront, for it is a constant reminder that there are more things in heaven and earth than are dreamt of in allopathic philosophy.

3

Why Does Homeopathy Work?

ANYONE INTERESTED in health and healing should try to answer this question: Why does homeopathy work?

That homeopathy does work is abundantly clear from many testimonials by both patients and doctors. I have described my own experience with it and mentioned some historical successes. I could list many more.

In a cholera epidemic in Europe in 1832, homeopaths had far higher recovery rates than regular doctors, with the result that the price of homeopathic medicine for cholera soared in Paris. Homeopaths were also successful in subsequent epidemics of scarlet fever, meningitis, and yellow fever.[1]

I have met elderly people who have had homeopaths as family doctors all their lives and have been so satisfied that they would not consider going to any other kinds of practitioners.

Homeopathic journals are filled with case reports of dramatic cures. Here is one example from 1952:[2]

> About two months ago a man in his forties came to my office. For six months he had made the rounds of dermatologists, visiting 7 or 8 of the best known men in New York and Brooklyn. Lotions, salves, oral medications, and injections had all been tried without result. At all times he wore white cotton gloves because the reddish-brown eruption on both hands emitted a foul odor and watered constantly. At least 3 or 4 daily changes of gloves were necessary, and he feared to approach his clients because of the condition of his hands ... He feared loss of his mind and contemplated suicide.
>
> Careful questioning did not reveal any marital discord although

he admitted a lack of interest in sex. Venereal disease was denied, both personally and in his family . . .

In spite of the denial of luetic [i.e., syphilitic] history and report of negative tests by previous doctors, the patient's exhaustion and emaciation, the mental picture, and the need for alcoholic stimulation, together with the modalities, made me decide on *Syphilinum* as the remedy of choice.*

The patient had never had homeopathic treatment previously and was therefore warned that the drug he was to receive was a very potent one and might cause him to become much worse within 12 to 36 hours . . . It was most fortunate that I had so impressed him, for as he related to me a week later, he felt dreadful about 18 hours after taking the remedy. Fluid poured from his hands at such a rate that he could not wear gloves, and the burning became intense. He became frightened and would have sought other attention had he not remembered my telling him that a severe reaction would be followed by a quick cure. After six hours of intense suffering, relief set in, and in one week there was hardly any evidence of the dreadful disease he had had. In the almost two years since his recovery there has been no return of symptoms.

Several homeopaths have told me of successful cures of acute pneumonias by Hahnemannian technique alone. One described the difficulty he experienced as a student of homeopathy when confronted by a case of pneumonia that seemed to demand aggressive antibiotic therapy. His allopathic training argued for penicillin, but his preceptor recommended close observation and a single dose of Pulsatilla, a dilute preparation of a species of windflower. Although he could hardly imagine withholding penicillin in such a case, he followed the homeopathic recommendation, and the patient recovered smoothly. The man has since rejected allopathy to practice exclusively as a homeopath.

Stories of this sort require us to take homeopathy seriously. Nevertheless, allopaths have long tried to dismiss such case histories as meaningless. Oliver Wendell Holmes took just that position in his 1842 attack. He wrote that the fact of homeopathic cures should not be admitted as evidence, because 90 percent of cases commonly seen by a physician "would recover sooner

Syphilinum is a homeopathic remedy prepared from scrapings of a syphilitic chancre.

or later, with more or less difficulty, provided nothing were done to interfere seriously with the efforts of nature."[3] In other words, most sick people will get better no matter what you do to them as long as you do not actively make them worse.

This is a strong argument, consistent with the experience of most observers of illness. We may quibble over the percentage of cases that will recover anyway, but it is certainly high, and may well be 90 percent. How, then, can we evaluate the effectiveness of *any* medical treatment?

Holmes's argument goes right to the problem of cause and effect. When two events, A and B, occur together in time such that B usually follows A, we tend to say that A causes B. That is just an interpretation, however. We cannot know in an absolute sense that A causes B, even if we come up with many logical reasons why it should be so.

Scientists try to build up confidence about cause-and-effect interpretations by means of experiments. Do A over and over in a laboratory and observe B happening regularly: A causes B. Unfortunately, medical treatments do not lend themselves to clean experiments. A sick person is a particular individual in a particular physical state at a particular time. He or she will never be exactly the same again, making an exact repetition of an experimental treatment impossible. Patients who recover from pneumonia after taking homeopathic remedies are unique. We cannot repeatedly make them sick with pneumonia and repeatedly give them the remedies to see if they will always recover.

It is possible that homeopathic treatment causes the many cures observed to follow it. If so, we might well ask how it does so. It is also possible that homeopathic treatment does not cause subsequent cures. Maybe the patients would have recovered anyway. We will never know.

Moreover, there is a third possibility to consider. Perhaps homeopathic treatment causes cures but not for the reasons homeopaths think. The mere act of treatment, independent of its content, can elicit cures by means of the placebo response.

The possibility that a treatment works as a placebo rather than a direct cause of improvement bedevils medical research. Doctors are always trying to rule out placebo effects, lest they draw incorrect causal relationships and endorse worthless treatments. Let me recount the saga of one such blunder.

Angina pectoris is pain in the chest on exertion — a dramatic symptom of coronary artery insufficiency. In coronary disease, blood supply to the heart is reduced; during exertion the shortage of blood can become so severe that the heart muscle starts to hurt. Doctors call it *ischemic* pain, meaning "from lack of blood." People suffering angina attacks usually stop whatever they are doing and stand still or sit down until the pain stops. They also commonly put nitroglycerine tablets under the tongue, since that drug dilates arteries, reducing the heart's workload and increasing its blood supply. Angina is a serious symptom, often worsening over time, and often predicting future heart attacks, in which portions of heart muscle actually die from lack of blood.

Although angina is a subjective complaint, there are ways of documenting it objectively and estimating its severity. Frequency of attacks and nitroglycerine requirement are useful criteria, as is capacity for effort. To measure effort capacity, patients are asked to walk up and down a two-step platform until chest pain begins. This test can also be done while recording the electrocardiogram to look for abnormal changes on exertion; it is then called the "Master 2-step test" after its inventor, a cardiologist named Arthur M. Master.

In 1957 an investigator named Cesarman working at the National Heart Institute in Mexico City made an accidental discovery that indicated a hopeful possibility for angina sufferers. He was using a new drug called iproniazid, a so-called "psychic energizer," to treat depressed psychiatric patients. It happened that some of the patients had angina. Cesarman noticed that their chest pains went away when they started taking iproniazid.

This chance observation led him to give the drug to a larger group of patients with angina. He reported the results in a paper titled "Serendipity and Angina Pectoris," published (in Spanish with an English summary) in the *Archivos del Instituto de Cardiología de Mexico*.[4] In it he wrote: "The action of iproniazid was studied in 41 patients with severe, intractable angina pectoris. The clinical manifestations of angina disappeared in all . . . It is believed that iproniazid is a specific drug for the treatment of angina pectoris."

Cesarman's paper led another investigator named Cossio in Buenos Aires to test iproniazid on thirty-six patients with angina. Cossio gave them 25 to 50 milligrams of the drug every eight hours for three to six weeks, recording frequency of attacks, need for nitroglycerine, and electrocardiogram at rest and during the Master 2-step test. His results, published in *La Prensa Medica de Argentina*,[5] also in 1957, showed disappearance of pain in 40 percent of patients, marked improvement in another 30 percent, and no change in the remaining 30 percent. There was no change, however, in the electrocardiogram of any of the subjects. Cossio concluded:

> These results are explained by a selective action of the drug on muscular pain of ischemic origin rather than on coronary vaso-dilatation or reduction of the work of the heart.
>
> Side effects, which were never serious but only troublesome, were reversible by suppression of the drug for a shorter or longer period, and administration could be resumed later in smaller doses.
>
> There are well-founded hopes that iproniazid is an important acquisition in cardiovascular therapy. It is believed that with more experience in this field, and perhaps with other methods of administration and higher doses, the percentage of unsuccessful cases will diminish.

These two reports from Latin America soon came to the attention of the leading North American expert on angina, Arthur M. Master, who was inspired to test the drug himself. He published his results in the *American Heart Journal* in October of 1958.[6]

Master summarized his findings as follows:

> Seventy-four patients with severe angina pectoris were treated with iproniazid, beginning with 150 milligrams daily, for from 1 week to 5 months.
>
> In my long experience with innumerable drugs for coronary disease, not one has approached the subjective relief attained by iproniazid.
>
> In more than one half of the patients, 41 to be exact, iproniazid relieved the anginal syndrome completely or almost completely . . .
>
> Neither the resting electrocardiogram nor the Master "2-step" test was altered during the course of treatment with iproniazid, indicating that the fundamental coronary disease was not altered, at least in this 5-month period.
>
> The precise mechanism of the relief of pain by iproniazid is

unknown. It can possibly be explained by cerebral stimulation, with uplift of mood, and increase of the pain threshold. There may be a direct effect on the autonomic nerve connections between the heart and the spinal cord and brain.

Unlike Cesarman and Cossio, Master noted severe side effects of iproniazid, including sudden falls in blood pressure that led to dizziness and fainting. Patients complained of stomach and urinary symptoms. Several developed peripheral nerve inflammation and weight gain. One got hepatitis. Mental symptoms, such as euphoria and excitement, were common. As a result, Master recommended close supervision of angina pectoris patients receiving iproniazid as well as efforts to find analogs of the drug with lower toxicity.

One may imagine the effect of this paper. For the foremost expert on angina to state in a leading journal that he had never seen anything comparable to iproniazid for the subjective relief of anginal pain was tantamount to a call to use the drug despite its dangerous side effects. As a result, research on iproniazid and analogs of it increased.

None of the studies mentioned here and none of those that immediately followed them were carefully controlled. That is, the investigators had no way to know whether pain relief was a direct effect of the drug or a placebo response to the mere act of giving a pill. As it happens, anginal pain is very responsive to placebo treatment, making controlled experiments absolutely necessary.

Not until 1961 were the results of such experiments published.[7] This time the drugs were administered in double-blind fashion. That is, neither the patients nor the doctors knew which patients got real drugs and which got inert sugar pills. Only at the end of an experiment, after the results were in, was that information revealed.

The controlled experiments showed iproniazid and its relatives to be *less effective than sugar pills* in relieving the pain of angina. They brought to an end this embarrassing episode in allopathic clinical medicine and spared future angina patients the hazards of taking drugs that could do real harm but could not help their illness by any pharmacological process. In the light of this clear-cut finding, it is interesting to go back and read the papers of Cesarman, Cossio, and Master to get a sense of the danger of relying on uncontrolled observation to draw cause-and-effect relationships between treatments and cures.

I do not wish to go further into the matter of placebos here. I will state my belief that we can never rule out placebo effects, no matter how carefully we control our experiments or how blind we make them. The reason is simply that placebo effects are products of the mind, and we can no more separate them from direct effects of drugs than we can separate mind from body.

Returning to the problem of why homeopathy works, we cannot exclude the possibility that Hahnemann's remedies are good placebos. Certainly they are not harmful, like an allopathic dose of iproniazid, but are they any more responsible for disappearance of symptoms than iproniazid in cases of angina? Homeopaths, of course, are very resistant to the idea that their remedies are placebos, especially since allopaths have long accused them of giving drugs with no more intrinsic effectiveness than sugar. They argue that their remedies produce real and dramatic effects, even in children and animals, who, they would have us believe, are incapable of responding to placebos.

Controlled studies of homeopathy are almost nonexistent. A 1980 report in the *British Journal of Clinical Pharmacology* evaluated homeopathic therapy in patients with rheumatoid arthritis.[8] All patients were on orthodox anti-inflammatory drugs. Some received homeopathic remedies in addition, while others got inert substances as controls; neither doctors nor patients knew who got what until the experiment was over. At the end of three months of observation, the investigators concluded that the addition of homeopathic treatment produced significant improvement of rheumatoid arthritis. This study is noteworthy because it took place in an allopathic institution as a collaborative project between regular doctors and homeopaths. It is one piece of evidence for some intrinsic activity of homeopathic remedies, but it cannot lay the placebo issue to rest.

What of the possibility that homeopathic medicine works as its practitioners believe? The Law of Similars is not difficult to accept. It makes as much sense as any other treatment rationale and even operates in a limited way in orthodox medicine. Vaccination is a form of similar treatment, for example, as is allergy desensitization. Some specific drugs now used by regular doctors were first brought into therapeutics by homeopaths. Nitroglycerine, the standard remedy for relief of anginal pain, was introduced into medicine by Dr. Constantine Hering (1800–1880) of Philadelphia, known as the father of American homeopathy. Based on his provings of this compound, he began treating angina and other heart conditions with it in the early 1850s, publishing his results in 1857. No mention of allopathic use of nitroglycerine for angina occurs until 1882. Allopathic use of metallic gold in the treatment of rheumatoid arthritis dates back to 1935; well before that date, homeopaths prescribed it for arthritis, because in the provings it produced a range of rheumatic symptoms.[9]

It is the Law of Infinitesimals that sticks in the throats of regular doctors and has caused generations of scientifically minded writers to dismiss homeopathy as nonsense, whether it cures people or not. The problem scientists have with this law is very clear.

Table salt is a compound of one atom of sodium (atomic weight 22.99) and one atom of chlorine (atomic weight 35.46). One molecule of sodium chloride has a molecular weight of 58.45, and one mole of sodium chloride is the molecular weight in grams: 58.45 grams, or about two ounces. That amount of salt dissolved in a liter of water forms a solution of standard concentration known as a molar solution. Count Amadeo Avogadro (1776–1856), an Italian chemist and physicist who was a contemporary of Samuel Hahnemann, calculated the number of molecules in one mole of any substance: 6.0225×10^{23}, a figure known to chemists and physicists today as Avogadro's number. According to Avogadro's calculation, one liter of a molar salt solution contains 6.0225×10^{23} molecules of sodium chloride. One liter of any molar solution contains that same number of molecules of the dissolved substance.

If we make serial dilutions of a molar salt solution, in the manner of preparing a homeopathic remedy, we can calculate how many molecules of salt remain at each level of dilution. Dilutions beyond the range of 10^{-24} will be unlikely to contain even a single molecule of sodium chloride. This is the Avogadro limit. The initial tinctures that homeopathic pharmacists begin with are at or near the molar concentration (Avogadro's number of molecules per liter), and the dilutions they prepare go well beyond the Avogadro limit.*

Attacks on homeopathy by scientists have ridiculed this aspect of the system. Why not put a drop of homeopathic medicine in Lake Erie, scoffed one doctor in the 1800s, and turn the whole lake into a vast therapeutic reservoir?† Homeopaths go through interesting contortions to counter these criticisms, and I want to summarize their case.

In the first place, they say, many homeopathic drugs are used in concentrations on this side of the Avogadro limit. That is all well and good, but the fact is that many homeopathic drugs are also used in concentrations far beyond the limit. The dose of sulfur I received on my visit to Berkeley was taken from a 200C dilution. It is not uncommon to encounter homeopathic preparations in dilutions of 1000X, 20,000X, or even 100,000C!‡

Moreover, the Law of Infinitesimals says the higher dilutions will be the stronger remedies. A contemporary homeopath writes:[10]

> How do we actually know that the therapeutic power of potencies truly increases with further dilution and succussion? This is confirmed by the frequent clinical observations of all homeopaths. Once the correct remedy is selected according to the Law of Similars, it is true that it will act even in crude form. For example, a patient with a Belladonna fever (with all the individualizing homeopathic symptoms found in the provings of Belladonna), will repond to even just a few drops of Belladonna tincture. The response may be minimal, however, and short-acting. If a 12X potency of Belladonna is given, the relief will likely be more dramatic. If, however, we administer a 10,000C potency, the response

*Dilutions in homeopathic shorthand are designated in two systems, written "X" (for powers of 10) and "C" (for powers of 100). A one-in-ten dilution, written 10^{-1} in chemical shorthand, is known as 1X in homeopathy. One part of that in ten volumes becomes a one-in-a-hundred dilution, symbolized 10^{-2} or 2X. Using the "C" notation, this same 2X dilution can also be abbreviated 1C. The next step is one-in-a-thousand: 10^{-3} or 3X. The 10^{-4} preparation is 4X or 2C, and so on. Any dilution higher than 24X or 12C is beyond the Avogadro limit. The chances that it contains even a single molecule of whatever substance the homeopathic pharmacist started out with are vanishingly small.
†The homeopathic rejoinder to this argument would be that such a vast reservoir does not constitute a remedy because it is not prepared by the Hahnemannian method of serial dilutions with succussion in between.
‡These numbers represent exponents — powers of 10 and 100 (see footnote above); 20,000X is almost inconceivably far beyond the Avogadro limit.

will likely be a complete disappearance of all symptoms within a matter of hours, with no relapse whatever.

The next rejoinder from homeopaths is that orthodox scientists have no evidence for rejecting the possibility that high dilutions of substances can have significant effects. This is true. Most allopaths and chemists just say that "common sense" tells us there is no difference between a 200X dilution and the plain alcohol-and-water mixture used as the solvent. Homeopaths do not want to hear about common sense. They want to see experimental evidence.

In an effort to bolster their claims, they have looked for examples of powerful effects of very dilute forms of biologically active substances. Many such examples exist, some having come to light only in recent years. Thyroid hormone circulates in the blood at a concentration of one part in 10,000 million (10^{10}) parts of plasma, yet controls general metabolism. Lysergic acid diethylamide (LSD) produces major changes in consciousness in doses as low as a few millionths of a gram, making for very low concentrations of LSD molecules in body fluids. Penicillin in 10^{-9} dilutions can inhibit the growth of certain sensitive bacteria. Some plant hormones cause spectacular increases in growth when applied in equally low concentrations. Even more impressive are the olfactory hormones, or pheromones, of insects, such as the sex attractants of certain moths. They may be the most potent biologically active compounds known in terms of how few molecules per volume of air are necessary to guide male moths to a receptive female.

There is, then, ample and growing evidence of the power of very dilute forms of certain substances to influence physiology and behavior of plants, animals, and humans; however, "very dilute" is not "extremely dilute." There is an enormous difference between a 10^{-9} or 10^{-10} dilution and a homeopathic 30X or 300X dilution. The former contain significant numbers of molecules of original compounds, and the effects we see are due to those molecules. The latter probably contain no molecules of original substances, so that if they exert effects on animals or human patients, they do it in some other way.

Homeopaths next point out that some research is on record

documenting physiological effects of dilutions beyond the Avogadro limit. This is also true, but it is not likely to impress critics, because what there is of it is exclusively the work of homeopaths, published in journals not read by physicists, chemists, and allopathic doctors. I will not attempt to summarize it here but will give one example.

In 1930 an investigator named Persson, working in Leningrad, studied the effects of dilutions up to 10^{-120} on enzymatic reactions. In one experiment, the substance tested was mercuric chloride, prepared in various dilutions. It was added to flasks containing identical mixtures of a starch solution and the salivary enzyme ptyalin, which converts starch to sugar. Control flasks contained only distilled water, starch, and ptyalin with no added mercuric chloride. Persson carefully measured the amount of sugar produced in each flask at a standard time after beginning the test. He found that mercuric chloride affected the rate of conversion of starch to sugar even in dilutions as high as 10^{-120}. No variations were observed in the control flasks. Results of these experiments appeared in the *Journal of the American Institute of Homeopathy*.[11]

Between 1946 and 1952, William Boyd in Edinburgh ran exhaustive repetitions of Persson's work, using mercuric chloride in dilutions up to 10^{-61} and paying scrupulous attention to technique, controls, and statistical analysis of results. In 1954 he published his findings in the *British Homeopathic Journal*.[12] In his summary, Boyd wrote: "All the series gave a highly significant difference in the rate of hydrolysis [i.e., the conversion of starch to sugar] between controls and tests, the microdoses stimulating the process . . . The solutions were theoretically 'dilutions' of the order of 10^{-61} and on present physical theory would not contain any molecules of the original mercuric chloride."

If impartial researchers can replicate these results according to the best methods of modern biochemistry — a big "if" — they will disturb the foundations of orthodox science. What possible mechanism can explain the biochemical and physiological actions of substances diluted beyond the Avogadro limit?

Contemporary homeopathic theorists have proposed one mechanism. They say previous presence of molecules of a substance in a solution diluted by Hahnemann's method (that is, with succussion between each dilution) might somehow change the molecular structure of the solvent in a permanent way, so that even if no drug molecules are left, the liquid is not the same as liquid that did not undergo the process. Both may be nothing more than an 87 percent solution of alcohol in water, but one carries some sort of "imprint" of the substance passed through it.

The nature of this imprint is unclear, even to those who propose it. Is it electrical? Or a spatial rearrangement of alcohol and water molecules into new patterns? Homeopaths do not know.

Here is the essence of an unreconcilable philosophical difference between allopathy and homeopathy. Regular doctors give drugs because they value properties attributed to the substance of those drugs. It is the *material* aspect of a drug that counts. Homeopaths use remedies containing no drug materials, yet they believe in the existence and therapeutic power of some other aspect of the drug — of its idea, if you will, or its ghost or spirit. Truly, homeopathy is spiritual medicine, consistent with its founder's views on the relative importance of spiritual versus material reality.

In attributing effects to dilutions of drugs higher than 24X and refusing to concede that these remedies function as placebos, homeopaths are asking us to create new physical and chemical laws, to rewrite accepted scientific theory — nothing less. Scientific theory does not change easily or without good reason. Even with good reason, the process is slow and painful.[13]

Challenges to science usually take form as anomalies that cannot be explained by current theoretical models. Champions of change make much of these anomalies to support their demands for revisions. Conservatives try to explain away anomalies with existing theory or to ignore anomalies they cannot explain. If anomalies become important enough or numerous enough, tension between proponents and opponents of the orthodox view may build to the point of a true scientific revolution that will result either in vindication of the existing theoretical model (and an end to the challenge) or its overthrow in favor of a new one with better explanatory power.

Is the fact of homeopathic medical success enough of an anomaly to bring about a scientific revolution? I doubt it. In the first place, most scientists and doctors are ignorant of homeopathy and have no sense of the theoretical challenge it poses. Second, it is too easy for orthodox M.D.'s to explain away homeopathic cures as placebo responses or as patients' getting better anyway.

We have looked at three hypotheses to explain why homeopathic treatment works. The first was that it works only because most patients will recover anyway, the treatment being irrelevant. Unfortunately, we can never know whether a given patient would have recovered anyway. The second hypothesis was that homeopathic remedies work by eliciting placebo responses. The problem with that one is the impossibility of ever cleanly separating placebo effects from direct effects of treatments.* The third hypothesis was that homeopathy's own explanation of its successes is valid, but as I have just shown, acceptance of it requires major revisions of basic physical and chemical theory.

None of these hypotheses is satisfactory, and there is no way to decide among them. Maybe all of them contribute to the right answer, if there is an answer.

I raise the question of why homeopathy works early on in order to draw the dimensions of my subject. Health and healing are of utmost concern to all of us, yet no matter how much scientific thought is directed at them, they remain partly mysterious. Sickness raises very practical questions. Why do we get sick? What should we do to get well? How do we avoid getting sick again? I intend to look for practical answers to these questions, not by summarizing medical science or listing recipes for the treatment of common ailments but by examining the concepts of health, disease, treatment, healing, and cure so that readers will be able to make informed decisions about the bewildering array of therapeutic choices available.

*See chapters 19 and 20.

II

WHAT IS HEALTH?

4

Health as Wholeness;
Wholeness as Perfection

WE KNOW HEALTH WELL in its absence.

When we are sick or injured we have no trouble knowing how things should be. A pain should not be there. An arm should move freely. A rash should go away. "Freedom from disease" is a common dictionary definition of health. Since *disease* comes from an Old French word meaning "lack of ease," we are left with a doubly negative sense: health is the absence of an absence of ease.

It ought to be possible to describe positively a concept so important to us. We talk about our health much of the time. (Some people talk about it most of the time.) We spend a great deal of money trying to restore or improve it. We join health clubs, visit health resorts, buy health foods. Yet in my years of formal medical education I never heard a good answer to the question, "What is health?" When I ask people to define health without using a negative construction, they often cannot.

The concept of health is at once simple and subtle. It is difficult to define only because we are no longer used to thinking about ourselves in the necessary philosophical terms. For example, medicine, religion, and magic are rooted in common ideas, and each sheds light on the others, but the supremacy of scientific technology makes it fashionable to believe that medicine has nothing to do with such old-fashioned practices as religion and magic. Consequently, many modern doctors cannot grasp the true meaning of health and can only define it negatively as freedom from disease. What the word really signifies is much more interesting.

I intend to delve into the realm of philosophy and symbolism to clarify the concept of health. I will examine some deep and perhaps unfamiliar ideas and will ask the reader to bear with me. These ideas are fundamental to the practical discussions of treatment coming later. Whenever possible, I will give concrete examples in order to show their relevance.

The root meaning of *health* is "wholeness." The word comes from the same Anglo-Saxon root that gives us *whole*, *hale*, and *holy*.

Cure and *care* come from one and the same Latin root: to cure is to take care of. *Treat* has a similar root meaning in Old French: to deal with or manage toward some particular end. *Medicine* comes from Latin *medicina*, and that word derives from an ancient Indo-European root that has also given us *remedy*, *meditate*, and *measure*. The root seems to suggest "thoughtful action to establish order." Thus *cure*, *treatment*, and *medicine* all suggest action to restore some aspect of wholeness implied by the word *health*.

What are the special properties of wholes that unite and animate such powerful concepts as health and holiness? If the answer to that question were obvious, we would have no need of redundant phrases like "holistic health."

Two properties of wholes command attention. By definition wholes are complete and perfect; they lack nothing. Moreover, in an ideal whole, the components are not only all there, they are there in an arrangement of harmonious integration and balance. Perfection and balance are traditional attributes of holiness. They also underlie the concept of health.

All religions see the ultimate reality as utterly perfect, all-encompassing. Nothing can exist apart from it. As the Great Whole, it is the origin of holiness in the world. Hinduism calls that reality Brahman, pure Being, which includes the creative, preserving, and destructive aspects of existence. In Judaism it is That Which Was and Is and Shall Be, so holy that the Hebrew name for it cannot be written or pronounced, because language would limit it.

In practice, many religions have specified that persons wanting to approach the ultimate reality must reflect its perfection as much as possible. For example, the Old Testament gives a stark recitation of prohibitions about those who may lead worship (Leviticus 21:16–23):

> And the Lord said to Moses, "Say to Aaron, None of your descendants throughout their generations who has a blemish shall draw near, a man blind or lame, or one who has a mutilated face or limb too long, or a man who has an injured foot or an injured hand, or a hunchback, or a dwarf, or a man with a defect in his sight or an itching disease, or a scab or crushed testicles; no man of the descendants of Aaron the priest who has a blemish, he shall not come near to offer the bread of his God, both of the most holy, and of the holy things."

In other words, a priest of the holy God must be holy in his person. He must be intact, whole, *healthy*, reflecting the perfection of his Creator. This link between the holy and the healthy is the common ground of religion and medicine. In many cultures, the two have never been separate.

Native American medicine men are religious leaders as much as doctors, treating spiritual and physical ailments at one and the same time. They often speak of the Medicine Wheel as the basis of tribal health, drawing on the circle as a universal symbol of wholeness and perfection. One great medicine man who spoke very eloquently about this symbol was Black Elk, an Oglala Sioux, born in 1863. At the age of nine, during a severe illness, he had a vision that was to be the source of his healing ability in later life. In one sequence of it, he related, a "great Voice said: 'Behold the circle of the nation's hoop, for it is holy, being endless, and thus all power shall be one power in the people without end.' "[1]

At the end of his life, Black Elk told his story to a white historian, who recorded his words. Black Elk said:

> You have noticed that everything an Indian does is in a circle, and that is because the Power of the World always works in circles, and everything tries to be round. In the old days when we were a strong and happy people, all our power came to us from the sacred hoop of the nation, and so long as the hoop was unbroken, the people flourished. The flowering tree was the living center of the hoop, and the circle of the four quarters nourished it . . . Everything the Power of the World does is done in a circle. The sky is round, and I have heard that the earth is round like

a ball, and so are all the stars. The wind, in its greatest power, whirls. Birds make their nests in circles, for theirs is the same religion as ours. The sun comes forth and goes down again in a circle. The moon does the same, and both are round. Even the seasons form a great circle in their changing, and always come back to where they were. The life of man is a circle from childhood to childhood, and so it is in everything where power moves. Our tepees were round like the nests of birds, and these were always set in a circle, the nation's hoop, a nest of many nests, where the Great Spirit meant for us to hatch our children.[2]

Black Elk poignantly lamented his people's banishment to the square, U.S.-government-built houses of the reservations, a symbol to him of the breaking of the nation's hoop. "It is a bad way to live, for there can be no power in a square."[3] The breaking of the sacred circle introduces imperfection and spiritual sickness, a loss of wholeness.

If the Creator and Creation are perfect wholes, how can imperfection exist? Or, in other words, why is there evil in the world? That is the supreme question for all religions and philosophies, and it must be understood that the question "Why is there sickness?" is just another form of it. Sickness is the manifestation of evil in the body just as health is the manifestation of holiness. Sickness and health are not simply physical states that the methods of science will eventually analyze completely and make understandable. They are rooted in the deepest and most mysterious strata of Being.

The most profound holy persons and philosophers tell us that evil is merely apparent or that it is the necessary other side that completes the whole of Creation. Buddhists say that good and evil in the relative world are both included in the perfect pattern of a higher Good. The God of the Old Testament declares, "I am the Lord and there is none else. I form the light and create darkness; I make peace and create evil; I am the Lord that do all these things."[4]

The idea that wholeness and perfection result from accepting and including the dark aspects of existence, even sickness and death, is a powerful line of thought that runs through many systems of practical magic and esoteric philosophy. It is also represented by well-known symbols, like the Tree of Knowledge of Good and Evil, which stands with the Tree of Life in the Garden of Eden.

The yin-yang symbol of Taoism graphically expresses the truth of perfection attained by integration of complementary opposites. This symbol and the philosophy behind it gave rise to the theory and method of Chinese medicine. The founder of Taoism, Lao-tzu, wrote:

> "One who has a man's wings
> And a woman's also
> Is in himself a womb of the world."
> And, being a womb of the world,
> Continuously, endlessly,
> Gives birth;
> One who, preferring light,
> Prefers darkness also
> Is in himself an image of the world
> And, being an image of the world,
> Is continuously, endlessly
> The dwelling of creation . . .[5]

In the Western tradition, one of the best symbols of this same idea is the caduceus, or wand of Hermes, the familiar winged staff with its intertwined snakes.

Medical historians sometimes say that the caduceus should not be the doctor's emblem, that it became so by confusion with another symbol, the staff of Asklepios, a plain staff with a single snake coiled round it. Asklepios (or Aesculapius in Latin) was the patron god of physicians in ancient Greece. Both doctors and patients offered sacrifices to him, and the final recourse of the very sick was to go to his temple, called the Asklepieion. Snakes were sacred to Asklepios and so were allowed to roam his temples freely. The ritual of the Asklepieion was simple: the sick would lie down in the great hall, listen to the hymns of the priests, and wait for night. Then they would stay until the god appeared to them in dreams and gave advice.

It may be that the staff of Asklepios is a logical badge for the doctor, and even that the wand of Hermes got mixed up with it somewhere along the way, but I consider the caduceus a far more appropriate symbol, because it embodies an esoteric truth that must be grasped to gain practical control over the shifting forces that determine health and illness.

Hermes is the messenger of the gods, the conductor of souls through the underworld, evolved, we are told, from the role of the herald in primitive Greek life; the caduceus as his emblem of power is a glorified herald's wand, brandished aloft in ancient courts to gain the recognition of kings and the right to speak and relate news. Hermes is a most ambivalent figure in mythology. Outwardly male, he is really androgynous. He is the scintillating Quicksilver of winged feet and cap, who carries the word of the Olympian gods to earth below, but he is also the grave and mysterious hermit, muffled in a dark cloak, who presides over alchemy and secret knowledge: the guardian of "hermetic science."[6]

The talents of Hermes — his speed, knowledge, effectiveness, and ability to protect from evil — all depend on his practical use of one chief secret: that power flows freely when the complementary opposites of existence are woven into the perfect pattern. That pattern appears in the caduceus. The two snakes, spitting at each other at the top of the wand, are the light and the dark, good and evil, yang and yin. In the hand of Hermes their bodies form regular sine waves that fit together into the sign of infinity, of the continuous, endless creation of Lao-tzu. As the number "8" that same sign is another symbol of Hermes. A figure 8 is a twisted circle viewed on edge, with power surging around it in the form of a continuous sine wave. Eight is the number of rhythm and dynamism. The snakes that twine around the wand are not frozen. They are in dynamic motion.

The wand itself, crowned with wings, intersects the nodes of that serpentine infinity. It is the middle path, the midpoint between opposites, where all power resides and all change is possible. Wednesday is the day of Hermes (named for Woden, his Teutonic counterpart) because it is the midpoint of the week, yellow his color because it is the midpoint of the spectrum. Apollo may be the exoteric god of healing in Greek mythology, but Hermes is its esoteric patron, since he presides over the perfect union of forces that is health and holds the secret knowledge of restoring that union when it breaks apart.

Restoring that which is broken is the function of religion; the word means "to bind again." Religion is medicine of the soul: the same activity directed toward the same end but concerned with the spiritual realm rather than the physical body. Magic is also the same activity. In most societies throughout most of history, magic, religion, and medicine have been intertwined, practiced together, and seen as having a common origin. The shaman of tribal peoples in northern Asia and the Americas is the doctor of bodies, souls, and situations. He (or she) has learned to be a personal mediator between the everyday world and the "other world," leaving his body to commune with spirits and learn the specific causes of illness, the whereabouts of missing objects, the reasons for failures of crops.

In our society, the commonality of religion, magic, and medicine is obscured. Our medical doctors have narrowed their view to pay attention only to the physical body and the material aspects of illness. As a result, they cannot practice the healing magic of Hermes because they do not see or integrate the nonphysical forces that animate and direct the physical body. For the same reason, many doctors cannot come up with a better definition of health than "absence of disease." They do not grasp the concept of wholeness as perfection that is the root meaning of the word, nor realize that health and illness are particular manifestations of good and evil, requiring all the help of religion and philosophy to understand and all the techniques of magic to manipulate.

Science and intellect can show us mechanisms and details of physical reality — and that knowledge is surely of value — but they cannot unveil the deep mysteries. You cannot restore health in yourself or in others until you know in your heart what health is.

5

Health as Wholeness;
Wholeness as Balance

IN AN IDEAL WHOLE, the components are not only all there, they are there in an arrangement of harmonious integration and balance. Balance is the other aspect of wholeness that enters into the meaning of health.

The word *balance* comes from Latin *bilanx*, as it occurs in the compound *libra bilanx*, denoting a balance or scale (*libra*) for weighing, made of two (*bi-*) flat plates (*lanx*). The word *libra* will be familiar as a sign of the zodiac represented by such a balance, the only astrological sign associated with an inanimate object rather than an animal or human.

The sign of Libra is ruled by Venus, goddess of beauty and harmony, suggesting that beauty arises from the balanced arrangement of components. Saturn is said to be "exalted" in this sign, that is, to reach its highest expression. Since Saturn is known to astrologers as the Greater Evil or Greater Misfortune (Mars being the Lesser), representing everything inimical to life, that relationship bears scrutiny.

In the heavens, the planet Venus is the brightest object next to the moon. Its light is warm, soft, and radiant, easily stimulating associations of feminine beauty, love, and peace. By contrast, Saturn's light is pale and cold, and that planet moves ever so slowly, barely changing its position against the stars from month to month. It is the outermost of the visible planets known to the ancients; its great distance from us and the sun accounts for its apparent slowness in our sky. I can see how our ancestors came to associate it with time and old age, with skeletons and cold, and other evils.

One image of Saturn is Father Time, holding an hourglass to measure out our allotted span of life. The Greek name for this old god who devoured his own children was Cronus; from it we get the combining form *chrono-*, meaning "time" (chronometer, chronic, synchronous, and so on). Another image of this same force is the Grim Reaper: Death as an animated skeleton who cuts down life with his scythe. In medical astrology, Saturn rules the bones — the most fixed, material components of our bodies, the skeletons we carry around beneath our living flesh and that will endure when all else has decomposed. Saturn is the force of limitation, that which cuts off all that grows and opposes all expansion. No wonder it earns the title of Greater Evil.

Yet this same force is said to be exalted in Libra, the sign of balance. The suggestion of that statement is that balance and harmony result from correct placement and use of limitation. To put the snakes of the caduceus into the mystic infinity pattern, you must oppose their tendency to stretch further outward when they have deviated just far enough from the midline.

If all this seems too abstract, consider a concrete example. I once lived in a country house in Virginia. On one side of the house was a huge, climbing rose, much overgrown, that did not flower. A professional gardener advised me to prune it. In late fall, when the plant was dormant, I cut it back extensively and with some regret, because I do not enjoy cutting living plants. From the point of view of the rose, the pruning was surely a dreadful experience, an assault by the Greater Evil. The next spring, however, it flowered magnificently, with a profusion of red blooms over many months. I think that story illustrates the practical meaning of the cryptical astrological statement of Saturn's exaltation in Libra. (It is especially fitting, incidentally, that red roses are one symbol of Venus.)

Properly aligned, the forces of expansion and limitation show us the place of balance, from which we can glimpse the perfection of a higher reality. Balance is truly a mystery. Learn to stand on your head or to walk a tightrope, and you will experience the mystery. The balance point is nondimensional but quite real. At first you overshoot it grossly, then overcorrect and miss it again in another direction. Your movements are exaggerated and jerky, anything but harmonious. Eventually, you become conscious of the special point, if only momentarily while falling through it.

Soon you can stay in it for several moments, becoming familiar with the distinctive feeling of effortlessness it provides. Lose it even slightly, and you must put out tremendous effort to regain it, but when you are on target, there is no work to be done. You can just enjoy the grace of a magical zone where all external forces cancel out by virtue of precise arrangement, one against another. In balance there is stillness and beauty in the very midst of chaos.

This stillness and beauty at the heart of change is the magic of the hurricane's eye, of the moment of totality of a solar eclipse, and, indeed, of the very stability of the earth itself, whose motions on its axis, orbit, and path around the galaxy with the rest of the solar system are so complex that merely trying to imagine them makes one giddy. The equinoxes of the seasonal cycle are magical points, as are the moments of sunrise and sunset, the *equilibrated* times of day, when reflection and meditation are possible with least effort.

The word *equilibrium* contains that same Latin *libra*. It is the state an analytical balance seeks as its two pans seesaw gracefully around the zero in harmonious motion. When the pans end their coupled dance and come to rest, they are in equilibrium, in this instance a static equilibrium, especially if the balance is enclosed in a protective glass case to screen out disturbing influences. In more complex systems, equilibriums are not static but dynamic, forged anew from moment to moment out of constantly changing conditions.

Dynamic equilibrium is a formal concept in chemistry, where it describes certain kinds of reactions. If table salt and sulfuric acid are mixed, they react to form hydrochloric acid and sodium sulfate. In addition, the newly formed substances react with each other to form more sodium chloride and sulfuric acid, because this is a reversible reaction. Eventually, the rate of the forward reaction and the rate of the reverse reaction become equal, and chemists say that a state of equilibrium exists.

The rates of such reactions and the time required to reach equilibrium depend on the nature of the substances, their molecular concentrations and physical states, as well as on temperature, pressure, and the presence or absence of catalysts. Once equilibrium is reached, the concentrations of the reacting substances remain constant, but this situation is not static. Rather, the forward reaction and the reverse reaction are taking place at equal velocities, with compounds breaking apart and re-forming continuously. The equilibrium is dynamic, giving the appearance of rest, while based on constant change.

The balance of health is also dynamic. The elements and forces making up a human being and the changing environmental stresses impinging on them constitute a system so elaborate as to be unimaginable in its complexity. We are islands of change in a sea of change, subject to cycles of rest and activity, of secretion of hormones, and of the rise and fall of powerful drives, subjected to noise, irritants, agents of disease, electrical and magnetic fields, the deteriorations of age, emotional tides. The variables are infinite, and all is in flux and motion. That equilibrium occurs even for an instant in such a system is miraculous, yet most of us are mostly healthy most of the time, our mind-bodies always trying to keep up the incredible balancing act demanded by all the stresses from inside and out. Moreover, they do it dynamically, since equilibrium is constantly destroyed and re-created.

The achievement of balance adds an extra quality to a whole. It makes the perfect whole greater than the sum of its parts, makes it beautiful and holy, and so connects it to a higher reality. Health is wholeness — wholeness in its most profound sense, with nothing left out and everything in just the right order to manifest the mystery of balance. Far from being simply the absence of disease, health is a dynamic and harmonious equilibrium of all the elements and forces making up and surrounding a human being.

6

Nine Principles of Health and Illness

IDEAS AND SYMBOLS must have practical meaning if they are to help us maintain health and decide how to treat illness. From the concepts of health as wholeness, perfection, and balance, I derive nine principles that form the background for considerations of treatment. These principles are consistent with my own experience, especially with observations of sickness in myself and others.

1. Perfect Health Is Not Attainable

Our working definition of health — a dynamic and harmonious equilibrium of all the elements and forces making up and surrounding a human being — leaves out one crucial word: "temporary." The balancing act of health is temporary only, destined to break down so that it can be reestablished as the foundation it rests on changes.[1]

Change is the essence of life, and the body is subject to change in so many dimensions that, again, the complexity is unimaginable. Periods of breakdown of equilibrium are periods of relative illness between peaks of relative health. Perfect health is an impossibility in the relative world, and any person or system promising it is not to be believed.

"Periods of relative illness" does not necessarily mean being sick in bed, or going to a hospital, or having to call a doctor. Relative illness can be as minor as a headache, a lack of energy, a few hours of indigestion, a night of restless sleep, a tiny injury. In fact, the valleys between new equilibrations may be so small that some persons might not call them illness and others might not even notice them. We have all met people who tell us they have never been sick a day in their lives.* Everyone gets sick. Some do not notice it or define it as sickness or let it affect their daily routine, and, perhaps, those are good ways of dealing with such changes.

As an observational exercise, I have sometimes recorded the little day-to-day ailments I experience. Here is a sample of one week's record from several years ago, when I was living in the Catalina Mountains near Tucson, Arizona:

Sunday: Woke up lethargic, dull mental feeling. Somewhat anxious, tending to overeat out of nervousness. Got cactus spine in right foot while walking barefoot in the desert. Neck and shoulders stiff in the evening.

Monday: Slept poorly. Throat a bit scratchy. Two whiteheads appeared on upper back. Some intestinal gas and looseness of stools.

Tuesday: Sneezing for no apparent reason, but throat is back to normal. Some difficulty in concentrating on mental tasks. Scratched up after a hike.

Wednesday: Woke up full of energy but got sad and introspective toward the end of the afternoon. Noticed a slight crack in lower lip, which is a bit sore.

Thursday: Lip mostly healed but burned my tongue on hot tea. Nothing else to report.

Friday: Had vivid, disturbing dreams that I don't remember well. Feet cold. Upper left arm itches off and on but nothing visible; skin seems generally dry.

Saturday: Stuffy nose. Left knee stiff. Very thirsty most of the day. Difficulty in falling asleep.

The record goes on in much the same way for subsequent days. I submit it as an example of the perfectly normal changes human beings go through as their bodies and minds adapt to the changing stresses of daily life. I consider none of these complaints serious; certainly, they do not require outside help or major corrective action. They just occur, and I notice them. I recommend this practice to the reader as a way of becoming

---

*A woman friend points out that such people are all male. The female experience of monthly "sickness" leads to easier acknowledgment and acceptance of cyclic breakdowns in health.

familiar with one's shifting state of relative health and the kinds of normal changes that disturb it.

Such a negative statement as "perfect health is not attainable" need not be cause for pessimism. The very dynamic nature of health rules out any static condition, and dynamism means alternations of ups and downs. If a temporary state of health is doomed to end, it is only to give way to a better one that takes account of a new configuration of stresses. The other side of this principle is that disease should not be static either. Even when it is serious and productive of great discomfort, it should be a temporary phase of bodily readjustment to new conditions.

2. It Is All Right to Be Sick

Seeing sickness as a calamity and misfortune directed at oneself for some particular reason is all too easy, but it is not compatible with the view that illness is the necessary complement to health, nor does it help people deal with the practical problems of being sick.

I saw a patient incapacitated by a severe respiratory flu that made the rounds one February. This thirty-two-year-old woman was very independent and strong and proud of those qualities in herself. When I visited her, she was at home in bed with fever, pain, and cough on the second day of the illness. Her mental state was abnormal as a result of fever and general infection, but her anger at being sick came through despite those changes and was not a direct result of the flu. She hated being helpless, could not remember when she had last had to stay in bed sick, wanted me to tell her she would be up and around the next day (when it was clear to me she would not be), and generally was fit to be tied. Besides the anger, she was feeling guilt. This calamity must say something about *her*: she had failed in some way or the illness would not have occurred.

I think it is fine to regard relative sickness as undesired and to work with all effort and intelligence toward reducing its severity and duration. We must not reject it as something that should not happen, however, nor interpret it as any sort of statement about our worth as human beings. Sickness does not mean; it just is.

Sickness is the way to the next relative period of health, and one state cannot exist without the other, any more than day can exist without night. Anger and guilt about falling sick not only go together with impossible dreams about attaining perfect health, they also *interfere* with the process of reaching a new equilibrium. I will have much to say about the interactions of mind and body in the course of these pages. Anger and guilt are real energies that can be transmuted into real physical effects by nervous and hormonal alchemy. As such, they further complicate the body's job of readjustment and may extend the time necessary for it.

3. The Body Has Innate Healing Abilities

Healing comes from inside, not outside. It is simply the body's natural attempt to restore equilibrium when equilibrium is lost. Healing cannot be prevented from occurring (though it can be obstructed in its expression), nor can it be obtained from anyone or anything external. You are born with the power to heal because healing is an innate capacity of every person, as it is of every animal and plant, and, I suspect, of every created thing.

Listen to sick people and you will hear much talk of seeking cures, healers, and healing. Medicines and medicine men can sometimes catalyze a healing response or remove obstructions to it, but they never give you what you do not already have. The power to heal is your property and birthright, ready to go to work whenever changing conditions create a demand for it.

4. Agents of Disease Are Not Causes of Disease

Materialistic medicine, which has so obscured the philosophical origins of the concept of health, has also fostered dangerous delusions about cause-and-effect relationships between diseases and agents that transmit them. Germs are *agents* of disease. They directly produce the immediate symptoms in certain conditions that affect us. For example, an influenza virus can inflame the lining of the bronchial tubes, causing irritation and reflex cough. A malarial parasite, injected by a mosquito into the blood of a susceptible person, can multiply in red blood cells till the cells burst, releasing substances that cause the characteristic chills and fever of malaria.

What about that word *susceptible*, however? Not everyone exposed to the parasite gets sick with malaria. In some individuals it fails to develop, either because it is checked by the immune system or for one or more other reasons we may not understand. Not everyone who meets up with flu virus gets flu, probably also for many possible reasons. Agents of disease do not cause us to get sick. They are merely potential vectors of illness waiting for chances to do their mischief. Given a chance, they will do it. Chances come along because of the natural fluctuations of our cycles of relative health. At a time of impending breakdown of equilibrium, an agent of disease might find fertile ground in which to develop or might act as the straw that breaks the camel's back.

Agents of disease are all around us, not only in the form of viruses, bacteria, and parasites but as a multitude of potential irritants, such as carcinogenic chemicals, allergens, insects, toxic plants, and so forth. A person solidly equilibrated in a phase of relative health can often interact with these agents and not get sick. Since internal factors determine the nature of our relationships with them, the true causes of disease are internal. I think those causes are also nonmaterial, having to do with the necessity of episodes of disequilibrium, a necessity imposed by the nature of reality.

Forgive me if I repeat myself; this point must be stressed: external, material objects are never causes of disease, merely agents waiting to cause specific symptoms in susceptible hosts. Susceptibility may well involve physical and chemical changes in body tissues, but those changes are initiated in another realm.

This principle suggests other ways of thinking about prevention and treatment than those predominant in conventional medicine. Rather than warring on disease agents with the hope (vain, I suspect) of eliminating them, we ought to worry more about strengthening resistance to them and learning to live in balance with them more of the time.

5. All Illness Is Psychosomatic

This proposition will be a hard one, but the difficulty is semantic only. *Psychosomatic* is a dirty word, its meaning muddied by years of wrong usage. All it means is "mind-body," nothing more. It does not mean "unreal" or "not serious" or "not physical" or "fake," just "mind-body."

To say that all illness is psychosomatic is to say only that all illness has both physical and mental components. This is not to imply that the physical symptoms are directly caused by the mind. There is another word for that, *psychogenic.*

How could it be otherwise? Mind and body are the two poles of our being, the nonphysical and the physical, which cannot exist apart from one another. Mind and body completely interpenetrate one another. The only way they can be separated is verbally, and, God knows, people have done enough of that ever since they had language.

Materialistic doctors talk about the mind but do not really believe in it, or, at least, do not accord it the reality of a physical organ that can be measured, experimented upon, and removed. When such doctors refer to psychosomatic illness, they mean only *some* illness, like asthma or ulcer, and often they also mean illness that seems to them exaggerated or not very important. For good reason, patients resent the word, protesting, "My asthma is real!" if someone dismisses it as psychosomatic.* All illness is psychosomatic because we are mind-bodies, not just bodies. That fact must influence therapeutic strategies in managing disease.

6. Subtle Manifestations of Illness Precede Gross Ones

To quote Lao-tzu again:

> Men knowing the way of life . . .
> "Face the simple fact before it becomes involved.
> Solve the small problem before it becomes big."
> The most involved fact in the world
> Could have been faced when it was simple.
> The biggest problem in the world
> Could have been solved when it was small . . .[2]

---

*I have thought hard about discarding the term, since its meaning is now so distorted. I like it, though. It is a good, solid word that says just what it says, and I don't know a better. A friend suggests I use *somatopsychic*, to avoid the inaccurate connotations that have grown up. If I cannot get my meaning across, I will do that. For now, I will try my best to clean up the word *psychosomatic* and will ask readers to pay attention to it when it occurs.

This observation by an ancient Chinese sage embodies an understanding of the way things come into physical existence. They follow a universal wave form, developing from subtle beginnings to highest peaks, then passing on. For some, say lightning bolts, this course may be completed so fast relative to our rhythms that we experience them as instantaneous events without clear beginnings and ends. For others, like mountains, it may be so slow relative to our rhythms that we experience them as static and unchanging. Nevertheless, all creations start small and grow, including conditions of disease.

Failure to notice and recognize disease at early stages is one of the main reasons for its severity and stubbornness. The earlier you notice a medical problem, the less work will be needed to correct it, to modify its course so that its peak will not be so high and its duration not so long. The farther into its course a disease proceeds before therapeutic measures are applied, the stronger the measures need to be and the smaller their chance of succeeding.

As a medical student on a surgery rotation at the Peter Bent Brigham Hospital in Boston, I once saw a patient who brought this principle home to me. He was a man in his midtwenties, a bricklayer, who came to the outpatient clinic with a terrible infection of his right hand. The hand was swollen to twice normal size, discolored, tense, with infection spreading rapidly up the arm, causing fever and other systemic signs. That was a surgical emergency, requiring admission to the hospital, surgical drainage of the hand, and massive dosing with antibiotics. There was no choice.

As the man was being readied for admission, I asked him why he had not come in sooner. His answer was, "It didn't bother me until this morning." That was the real problem. An infected hand does not get to that stage overnight. It may get there fast, especially if resistance is low and invading germs are aggressive, but there is always a preceding stage when infection is localized and contained by the body's defenses. Local infections in a hand can be managed quite well without drastic measures: by disinfection and diligent hot soaks, for example, while making sure the patient rests and eats and drinks wisely.

Unless you learn to notice and be bothered by the early, subtle stages of illness, you will lose your chances of managing your body through its changing cycles by simple means and will find yourself more and more dependent on outside practitioners and the costly interventions of modern hospital medicine.

7. Every Body Is Different

On some levels human beings may be the same or, at least, more alike than different. We may share a collective unconscious and a common spiritual essence. On the physical level, however, individual differences are common and important. Except for identical twins, people look different from each other. Moreover, anatomical individuality does not stop at faces and fingerprints; it extends to internal anatomy. Variation in form of stomachs is as great as that of noses. These differences may render people more or less susceptible to particular diseases. Quirks of urinary anatomy, like extra ureters or abnormally low kidneys, increase the risk of kidney infections. Some variations in the branching of the coronary arteries may improve the chances of surviving heart attacks.

Bodies differ in function as well as form. People are biochemically unique, too.[3] Simple genetic differences allow some persons to taste substances and digest foods that others cannot taste or digest. It is quite true that one man's meat is another man's poison. For example, many species of wild mushrooms are considered toxic because they make many people very sick to their stomachs, but some persons can eat the same mushrooms without any ill effects and enjoy doing so. Biochemical individuality is one reason for variations in responses to drugs — a fact not much emphasized in medical teaching.

The truth that every body is different makes generalization risky about the benefits and hazards of foods, drugs, and medical treatments. Research on the health hazards of cigarette smoking is convincing, but not everyone who smokes heavily will get lung cancer or other respiratory disease. I meet men and women in their seventies and eighties who have smoked two to three packs of cigarettes a day since adolescence and appear to be in better respiratory shape than some younger people who do not smoke. They must have had strong constitutions and strong respiratory systems to begin with. Of course, it would be an error to generalize from their experience. Many others who smoke that much will certainly suffer for it.

Readiness to ignore individual differences and generalize from personal experience accounts for a great deal of the contradictory dogma that characterizes the health professions, a problem glaringly visible in disputes over nutrition and diet. In reviewing all the dietary regimens loudly proclaimed as "the only right way to eat," I have come across serious arguments against every category of food. If all were right, there would be nothing to eat. Of course, a right diet probably exists for each individual, but what is best for me might not be best for you and might not even be best for me a year from now. As a generalization, the perfect diet is a fantasy.

This way of thinking also casts doubt on the universal applicability of any one form of treatment, whether it be drugs, surgery, acupuncture, massage, or any other procedure applied to the physical body. There is probably a best treatment for any individual with a particular problem, but, again, what is best for me might not be best for you even if our problems appear similar. As a generalization, the universal treatment or the perfect system of medicine is as much a fantasy as the perfect diet.

8. Every Body Has a Weak Point

Physical systems such as the human body are never like Oliver Wendell Holmes's Wonderful One-Hoss Shay* that, after a hundred years, finally fell to pieces all at once because every part was as strong as every other. Bodies have one or more weak points. It is useful to know those points because they tend to register stress as early warnings of impending breakdowns of health.

My throat is a reliable early-warning system. When I am low in energy, overstressed, and susceptible, my throat begins to feel rough, then sore. If I catch the change very early, I can usually both avoid a really sore throat and make sure I get back in balance, for example, by cutting down on nonessential expen-

*Described in the poem "The Deacon's Masterpiece, or The Wonderful One-Hoss Shay," from 1858.

ditures of energy, adjusting my intake of food and drink, and paying more attention to my physical, mental, and emotional needs.

Some people have sensitive stomachs that give them the same message, others irritable bladders or weak joints. Learn your weak points. They will give you signals when you approach periods of susceptibility to disease. Practice at recognizing those signals will help you notice illness in its subtle stages and improve your chances of correcting it by simple measures.

9. Blood Is a Principal Carrier of Healing Energy

Healing may be a nonmaterial energy rooted in the ultimate mysteries, but it makes use of perfectly familiar, physical mechanisms in trying to reestablish health. Blood is one of its main vehicles.

The worst scalp laceration, however ugly, dirty, and mistreated, usually heals uneventfully and speedily once it is washed and closed, even if sterile technique is not used. The reason is the rich blood supply of the scalp, one of the richest in the body.

At the opposite extreme is the foot of a patient with severe diabetes. Diabetes obliterates tiny arteries throughout the body, causing destruction of organs by cutting off blood flow to them. The lower extremities are frequent targets of this process, with the result that a diabetic's foot may receive only a fraction of the blood it needs. One consequence is enormously increased susceptibility to infection and decreased ability to heal. The slightest nick in the skin of such a foot may develop into an ulcer lined with dying flesh that refuses to heal and offers a perfect breeding ground for bacteria. Even with full medical support, an ulcer of this kind may become the focus of spreading gangrene that necessitates eventual amputation of the foot.

These two cases show very clearly the role of blood as a physical carrier of healing energy. A healthy circulatory system, with adequate and normal blood, is the keystone of the body's healing system. One of the most effective ways to promote healing, if it can be done, is to increase the amount of blood reaching an ailing part of the body.

*

I am sure there are other sound principles of health and illness that could be listed here, but these nine, with the philosophical considerations underlying them, will be sufficient to explore the questions about treatment that need to be asked: What is treatment? what should it be? when do you need it? and how do you go about selecting the kind of treatment that is best? I will discuss the nature of healing in somewhat greater detail, and then will address these very practical questions.

III
HEALING

7

The Nature of Healing

ANYONE WHO DOUBTS the body's ability to heal itself should pay attention to wound healing. It is a splendid way to learn the nature of the process and gain confidence in it as an innate capacity.

The next time you get a significant laceration or abrasion, try to detach yourself from the emotional upset of it as soon as possible. (Wounds are psychosomatic events, of course.) Then notice and record the changes that ensue. If there is pain, regard it as a correlate of the activity of nerves that are conveying information about the nature and extent of the injury to the brain and activating mechanisms for both immediate and long-term repair. Note its quality, duration, and change with time. If there is bleeding, see it as the body's way of cleaning the area and ensuring an unobstructed flow of blood.

Observe how bleeding stops with the formation of a clot. How soon can you detect the beginnings of an inflammatory response (redness, warmth, swelling, and tenderness around the injured tissue)? These changes represent the influx of white blood cells and other cells whose job is the removal of debris and defense against infection. Does a scab form? How long does it remain? Does itching occur? How does the scab come off? What is the appearance of the healed skin? Is there a scar? Or any loss of sensitivity or interference with movement?

Wounds are fascinating, and people have watched them, I suppose, ever since there were people. With the invention of writing, some people began to record their observations of wounds and their techniques of treating them. The methods that have come down to us in old writings are marvelous in their variety. Some seem sensible, some absurd.

Ancient Sumerians liked to wash wounds with beer and included beer as an ingredient in plasters. One prescription, on a clay tablet dated from 2100 B.C. and thought to be the world's oldest medical manuscript, says to pound together dried wine dregs, juniper, and prunes; pour beer on the mixture; then bind it on the wound after rubbing with oil. The oil might have served to prevent the plaster from sticking to the wound, and some of the ingredients might have antibacterial properties.[1]

Ancient Egyptian physicians put fresh meat on wounds, which may have promoted blood clotting, and they rubbed in many strange substances, among them the excrement of various animals and the powdered green mineral malachite. The role of dung in treating wounds is obscure, at best, but malachite turns out to be an effective germicide. It is copper carbonate, and copper salts are powerful antibacterial agents. Another favorite Egyptian wound dressing was a salve of honey and grease. Modern testing shows it to be a good antibiotic. Honey kills bacteria in several different ways and has been a folk remedy for wounds in many parts of the world, even into modern times.[2]

The list of substances recorded as wound treatments throughout history seems endless. A few of them may actually retard healing; most probably do nothing one way or the other. Some, like honey and malachite, may reduce the chance of infection. The fact is that most wounds heal with or without treatment. The only way to prevent a wound from healing is to infect it or leave foreign matter in it. Moreover, in thousands of years of experimentation, no one has found a way of speeding up the process of wound healing. In an otherwise healthy person, a wound that is clean and has bled freely will heal itself as efficiently as possible with no need of medicine, and we cannot make it heal any faster or better.

I find it interesting that the largest category of herbal remedies is the vulneraries, or wound healers. A great many plants are said to help wounds heal. The reason, of course, is that wounds heal, and if a plant does not actively interfere with the process, people will often come to see it as the cause of healing — the old problem of drawing cause-and-effect conclusions about medical treatments and cures.

Some plants feel good on wounds — the clear jelly in aloe

leaves is an example — and so may be soothing and welcome, but they do not speed healing. In my own investigations of botanical medicine, the most effective vulnerary I have come across is the latex of a Peruvian jungle tree (*Croton lechleri*). Peruvians call the sticky red liquid *sangre de grado*, a corruption of the Spanish name, "dragon's blood." Painted on a wound, it disinfects it, forms a tough, elastic skin that works better than a bandage, and seems to favor scab formation. Even this exotic remedy does not accelerate wound healing, however.

Disinfection of wounds should not be necessary if bleeding has occurred and there is no reason to think that unusual organisms have been introduced. If you must use a disinfectant, hydrogen peroxide is safest and best. It breaks down to ordinary water and an active form of oxygen that kills the most dangerous wound-infecting bacteria. Tincture of iodine, the standard and dreaded treatment of my boyhood, is a strong tissue irritant that probably adds insult to injury rather than does any good. The same is true of Merthiolate and mercurochrome; they are less irritating than iodine but equally useless. If these familiar substances have any influence on an uninfected wound, they may retard healing slightly. Experiment on yourself, and you will soon be convinced that ordinary wounds behave the same whether you disinfect them or not, subject them to stinging irritants, or anoint them with exotic and colorful herbs, salves, tinctures, and plasters.

Wound healing is a model for healing in general. Becoming familiar with it and understanding that it simply happens automatically and cannot be improved upon is an important piece of medical self-knowledge.

Wounds of the skin and superficial tissues heal rapidly compared to some other problems, even when they are extensive, as in abdominal surgery. A broken bone may take much longer to heal than a laceration. Lungs damaged by years of cigarette smoking may take very much longer. Also, some people heal faster than others — the young faster than the old, for example. Always, healing proceeds as best it can given the circumstances of its occurrence.

Healing is not just a property of the physical body. Remember: we are mind-bodies, so that healing, like health and illness, must also be psychosomatic. If injury or disease affects the mind primarily, then healing will take place in that realm.

Consider the psychic analog of wound healing — say the reaction to a severe emotional injury, such as the sudden death of a spouse or child. There is the same initial shock and intense pain that claims all attention and totally shatters one's equilibrium. There is a flood of emotion, perhaps the psychic analog of bleeding, and with time and normal grieving the gradual but steady development of scab and scar, the regeneration of positive feelings, and adaptation to the loss. The wound may ache on occasion, even years later, but it is then an old wound, a healed one, no longer a threat to equilibrium.

Healing involves several distinct components. Three that I distinguish are reaction, regeneration, and adaptation.

The inflammation that develops around the edges of a wound is an example of the reactive component of healing. Fever in response to infection is another, although most people regard it as a symptom of illness rather than an aspect of healing. That way of thinking leads most people (and not a few doctors) to treat fever as a problem to be reduced or eliminated, as by taking aspirin. Unless fever is dangerously high (over 105°F or 40.5°C), such action is probably unwise. There is clear experimental evidence that fever helps the body fight infection and that artificial lowering of fever gives invading germs an edge.[3] Reactive phases of healing may be dramatic and productive of discomfort, but it is important not to mistake them for primary symptoms of disease.

Regeneration is the most spectacular component of healing. Some of our cells and tissues have astounding regenerative ability. Liver cells can multiply fast enough to replace large portions of that organ within a matter of hours of their experimental removal.* Destroy the delicate cells that line the digestive

*This is a response of healthy liver cells to an experimental surgical procedure. In the world outside the laboratory, the liver is more vulnerable. Traumatic injury to it may result in fatal hemorrhage before cellular regeneration can repair the damage. Toxic injury from exposure to some chemical compounds can cause rapid death of the whole liver by deranging the metabolism of its cells. Unhealthy liver cells, such as those in alcoholic patients and victims of chronic hepatitis, lose their regenerative capacity and so cannot halt progressive destruction of vital liver tissue.

tract and cover many organs, and they will be replaced in a day or less.

I once had a chance to experience such regeneration in myself after a disabling episode of snow blindness. I went on an unplanned cross-country ski excursion high in the Colorado Rockies on a brilliant day in winter, lacking sunglasses. I was aware of the danger of snow blindness and made an effort to shade my eyes whenever I could; still, I underestimated the rapidity of sunburn at that altitude with such glare. I felt nothing but exhilaration from the trip when I arrived at the Grand Junction airport that afternoon to fly home to Tucson. An hour later, while waiting to change planes in Denver, I was overcome by tiredness and began to get a headache. My eyes felt sore and irritated, as if they had sand in them.

By the time I boarded the plane to Tucson, the soreness had increased so much that light bothered me, and my eyes started to tear. Shortly after takeoff, I had to close them. Then I drifted off into a brief, light sleep. When I woke up, I could not open my eyes. The slightest effort to raise the lids produced such intense pain that a muscular reflex took over and kept them tightly closed. I could not even pry them open. With the lids closed, my eyes felt raw and filled with grit, but these sensations were nothing compared to the searing pain that came with any attempt at opening.

I knew at once what the problem was, and since I also knew it would resolve spontaneously, I was not particularly worried; however, I could not remember how long snow blindness was supposed to last. I called a stewardess and explained my predicament. She brought me a cool cloth to keep over my eyes and seemed more upset than I. I told her my main concern was getting off the plane and into the airport, since I was completely helpless.

I had to be taken from the airplane in a wheelchair, much to the distress of the friend who came to meet me. I had never been so dependent in my adult life, nor blind ever — an educational experience indeed. I did not get home till late at night and went straight to bed, taking a sedative to help me sleep. By the time I began to get sleepy, I could already begin to open my eyes slightly and could detect the beginning of a decrease in pain and the sensation of irritation. The next morning I could open my eyes fully, although they still felt a bit tender. I wore sunglasses that morning but discarded them by the afternoon. In about twenty-four hours, my eyes were mostly healed. The following morning they felt perfectly normal.

Snow blindness results from a sunburn of the cornea, the transparent covering of the iris and pupil. The burned cells swell, die, and slough off, exposing tiny nerve endings that register intense pain and trigger reflex closing of the eyes. Within a day, a completely new layer of corneal cells can regenerate to replace the lost ones and protect the insulted nerves.

In lower animals, regeneration achieves results we cannot, such as replacement of whole body parts. Catch certain lizards by the tail, and the tail will come off in your hand, still thrashing, while the shortened lizard escapes. It will grow a brand-new tail promptly. Cut off the leg of a salamander, and a new one will regenerate.

Human beings seem to have the same potential to regenerate limbs and other organs, and researchers are trying to find out why they do not do it. Every cell of your body has in its genetic material all the information needed to make a new you, all of it coded in the molecular structure of DNA. Many cells, in addition, have the working machinery to turn that information into physical reality. In general, the more specialized a cell is, the less its capacity to regenerate itself or other tissues. Heart muscle is quite specialized, for instance, and when part of it dies, it is replaced by scar tissue rather than new muscle. Nerve cells in the brain are the most specialized cells of all and have no regenerative power; such a nerve cell lost is lost forever.

Limb regeneration in lower animals is organized by nerves, which seem to direct some cells at the wound site to *dedifferentiate*, that is, to lose their specialized identity as bone or cartilage cells and regress into general embryonic cells with the ability to make a whole range of tissues, including bone, cartilage, and all the other components of a new leg or tail. Since many of our cells have the same potential to dedifferentiate and regenerate missing tissues, we may one day find out how to grow new legs and hearts when we need them as easily as we can now grow new skin and corneal cells.

Regeneration will accomplish as much as it can in healing, but when it reaches a limit, another process must take over. The scar that forms in the heart of a heart-attack survivor is a healed area but not a regenerated one. The heart must adapt to the scar and compensate for the loss of a portion of muscle. In the first hours after a heart attack, the area of dead muscle is a focus of instability with potential to disrupt cardiac equilibrium (as by causing a sudden irregularity of heartbeat that can be quickly fatal). Healing by scar formation reestablishes stability, and the patient then can (and should) resume normal activity (perhaps with better habits of diet and exercise to minimize the chance of further losses of this nonreplaceable tissue).

Adaptation and compensation are important components of healing, when reaction and regeneration cannot completely reverse the destructive effects of injury or illness. The body adapts to its losses and finds the best way around them. In the case of a scarred heart, that may be the development of new circulation around the damaged area.

One kind of adaptive response is the isolation, or walling off, of a diseased area that cannot be returned to a healthy state. Such isolation may prevent the disease from affecting more of an organism. Just as oysters make pearls to protect themselves from irritating foreign particles, so our bodies can wall off pockets of infection to form abscesses. This process often occurs in tuberculosis of the lungs, where the body's defenses cannot defeat the infection but frequently can contain it. The end result is a cavity surrounded by a fibrous wall, with normal lung tissue beyond.

Adaptation goes on at the behavioral level as well as the cellular level. I know a middle-aged naturalist who, as a college student, was stricken with Guillain-Barré syndrome, a strange disease of the nervous system that mimics poliomyelitis and can cause the same kind of permanent disability by depriving muscles of their nerve supply. This man has lost considerable function of his legs, but his adaptation to and compensation for the loss are impressive. He is an active explorer of the world and gets around difficult terrain better than some unimpaired people I know.

Reaction, regeneration, and adaptation, like healing itself, are all automatic responses to the loss of healthy equilibrium. You do not have to think about them or work at them or seek them from outside. Healing just happens whenever the mind-body is disturbed. Indeed, it *must* happen, just as an analytical balance must react to being moved and must seek a new position of rest.

I mentioned in Chapter 6 that healing is probably a universal property of all creation. Certainly animals heal themselves, usually without benefit of medicines and doctors, and so do plants. I had the pleasure of living in a dense stand of giant sahuaro cactuses in southern Arizona for a number of years. Although their rhythm of life is slower than mine, living with them permitted me to watch them heal from injuries, reacting with a type of scar formation not so different from ours. I am ashamed to admit that I once caused injury to a sahuaro by building a bonfire too close to it. I thought the cactus was out of range, but the heat burned a two-foot section of the stem on the side facing the fire. The next day, the tough skin of the cactus turned pale in this area. In the following days it became paler still and softened, and I feared the plant would not survive, since the injured area could easily allow loss of water or entry of disease agents. It did survive, I am happy to say, and over the next year covered the damage with a thick scar of gray callous tissue, a barrier tougher than the original skin, if not as attractive. The cactus has grown normally since then.

Healing is not limited to what we call living things. I believe that rocks heal, too; their rhythms are just so slow compared to ours that we cannot see them change. The mountain range behind my house in Arizona was defaced while I lived there by a zealous builder who carved a zigzag dirt road up to his mountain retreat. The gouged line is visible from miles away. If we could watch that mountain with time-lapse photography over the next centuries, I am sure we would see the wound fade and disappear, much like a scratch on an arm. Its sharp contours would soften under the influence of weather and age, and vegetation would regenerate in the denuded area. Is there any reason not to call that healing?

When a distant star hurls a great chunk of itself into space in the huge explosion astronomers call a nova, the rest of the star quickly regains stability and equilibrium, rearranging its layers to cover the wound and continue the business of fusing matter into energy. Is there any reason not to call that healing?

I find these considerations helpful, because they emphasize the generality of healing, which is simply the universal tendency to seek equilibrium, a reaction to and compensation for any disturbance, using whatever mechanisms and materials are available.

Though healing is universal and innate and must occur in us in response to illness or injury, its results are sometimes inadequate. We have all seen injuries that do not heal, illnesses that do not end. What goes wrong when healing is incomplete or ineffective?

An obvious failure occurs when disturbing forces are so strong as to overwhelm an organism's ability to meet them and respond. Run into a person with an automobile at high speed, and death is a likely outcome. Deprive a plant of water and continue the deprivation long enough, and you will kill it.

There are men in India who smoke cobra venom regularly and eventually are able to let cobras bite them on the tongue. They say the venom gives a wonderful high, better than any familiar drug. This is certainly a curious practice and also a striking example of bodily adaptation. Alcoholics can swallow doses of liquor that would kill other people, because their systems have adapted to the regular presence of that poison. Still, there is some dose of cobra venom given all at once, and some dose of alcohol given all at once, that will overwhelm even the most adapted cobra guru or alcoholic, causing permanent loss of equilibrium. I am certain that most of us imagine our limits to be much more confining than they are, but limits do exist, including those that define the power of healing to restore lost balance.

Total inadequacy of a healing response to a disturbing force means death. More commonly, healing is partially inadequate, or, at least, unsatisfactory from the point of view of a sick or injured individual.

Return to the example of a wound. Wounds may fail to heal for a number of reasons. Healing energy may be unable to reach the site because of insufficient circulation to carry it there — the case of the diabetic's foot. Materials needed to repair the damage may be wanting, as in cases of malnutrition, especially protein deficiency. Healing may be opposed by destructive forces that aggravate the injury, such as infection.

A person with generally low vital energy may be unable to mount a sufficient healing response to repair a wound. The terminal cancer patient is an example, where vitality is sapped both by the cancer's derangement of total metabolism (resulting in the mysterious wasting known as cachexia), and by such treatments as radiation and chemotherapy, which weaken the blood-forming, immune, and digestive systems, all of which must be in good working order for effective healing to occur.

Finally, and most commonly, healing may be stalled or blocked. A simple mechanical problem may be the trouble. Once I injured my right foot badly while climbing barefoot on a slope of loose rock. I stepped on a big rock that split in two, one half of it falling on top of my foot and inflicting a deep laceration, about two inches long, just below the middle toes. It bled a great deal, but I was able to stop the bleeding with pressure and an improvised bandage and get home. Although I could see some exposed tendons, I knew there was no really serious damage and decided to avoid stitches. I just taped the edges of the wound together with adhesive strips. It closed as I expected, but within a short time reopened, discharging a little blood and watery fluid. There appeared to be no infection, but it would not heal.

I experimented with various dressings, the most bizarre (and messy) being the rind of a papaya, recommended by a neighborhood herbalist. None of them helped. Finally, after two weeks, the wound closed and seemed to be healing; it was a little sore but not a source of anxiety. A few days later, however, while I was soaking in a hot spring, it opened once again, looking the same as before: not infected but unwilling to heal. This time I went to a physician, who probed it at great length and after fifteen minutes came up with a chunk of rock the size of a pea. Within two days the wound healed completely and never gave further trouble. If anything, healing seemed accelerated, as if it had built up a kind of pressure or urgency in its frustration. That piece of foreign matter did not belong there, and it obstructed healing until removed.

If nerve fibers are severed, the portions beyond the cuts degenerate, but the portions attached to the nerve cells begin to regrow, albeit slowly, seeking their target organs.* A regenerating nerve fiber has a problem, though. It cannot get to where it is going unless it can enter the sheath that enclosed the previous fiber. More often than not, the severed ends of nerve sheaths are displaced when nerves are cut as a result of injury, and regenerating fibers cannot find the right sheaths to take them home. As a result, the muscles, glands, or other tissues beyond the cut are permanently deprived of their nerve supply and so cannot function normally. Healing happens but is thwarted by a simple mechanical problem.

In recent years, reports have become more and more common of surgical successes in reattaching severed fingers, hands, feet, and arms. This kind of surgery must be prompt, lest the severed appendage begin to die. The most delicate part of it is meticulous joining of nerve sheaths, so that regenerating fibers will reach their proper destinations. The regeneration may take weeks or even many months, depending on the distance that must be covered, but if the alignments are correctly made, full recovery of function will eventually come about.

A most dramatic and tragic form of nerve damage is spinal cord injury, often the result of accidents in otherwise healthy and athletic young people, who are rendered immediately paraplegic or quadriplegic, permanent invalids. Surgeons can repair the gross spinal injuries, removing bone splinters and blood clots, yet the vital nerve cord that carries messages to and from the brain and controls many muscles and organs remains obstructed at a certain level, even though the cord looks normal. In such cases, one can often observe a tendency to heal and reestablish function. For example, over the weeks or months following injury, sensation may return in border areas of the paralyzed zone, along with some motor activity. The nervous system seems to try to find new pathways of communication with the body, but usually any gains are very limited. Possibly, one day we will have the ability to assist spinal nerves in making new connections around cord obstructions resulting from injury.

Mechanical obstruction is one type of blockage of healing.

---

*It is nerve *cells*, especially in the brain and spinal cord, that cannot be replaced. Nerve fibers can regrow as long as the cells are intact.

Obstruction can be nonphysical as well, such as an interfering mental state. Strong anger, guilt, or anxiety focused on an ailing part of the body may prevent healing from reaching it as effectively as a physical barrier. I do not know the mechanism of this phenomenon but suspect it involves use of nerves by the mind in ways that limit their capacity to convey whatever they should convey for healing to occur.

Some systems of treatment are based on theories now discredited by medical science, yet they can elicit rapid cures even of serious conditions that have persisted over time. They seem to work mainly because people believe in them. If belief can be a key to unblock healing, it must also be able to block it. For every case of a wound that does not heal because a piece of foreign matter remains in it, there are probably many cases of disease that persists because the mind obstructs healing.

I do not think chronic disease is a simple matter of conscious choice or repressed emotion. It is not just that some patients stay sick because they derive what psychiatrists call "secondary gain" or that a man with ulcerative colitis cannot express anger at a parent or that a woman gets breast cancer because she has bottled up her feelings. Those simplistic formulations come nowhere near to portraying the intricacy and subtlety of the interplay of mind and body. That is the subject of a later chapter. For now, let me state my conviction that when healing is stalled or blocked, the source of trouble is likely to be in the nonphysical end of the human mind-body, and physical intervention will not lead to cure unless it also produces change in the mental realm.

The fact that healing can be blocked creates the possibility of treatment. We may not be able to improve on healing or speed it up beyond its own proper rate, but we can remove obstacles to it, supply it with missing materials, and help it reach a diseased site. It is a misnomer to call medicine "the healing art." The healing art is the secret wisdom of the body. Medicine can do no more than facilitate it.*

*I came across an eloquent expression of this truth in the motto of a social club I belonged to at Harvard Medical School, the Aesculapian Club: "We dress the wound, God heals it."

That is all healers can do, too. Many persons claim healing powers, and all sorts of professional healers offer their services, from faith healers and psychic healers to Indian medicine men. Some are frauds, some are genuine, but none put healing into anyone else. Good ones can remove obstacles to healing, motivate sick people to get well, and perhaps raise the vitality of debilitated persons in some way.

Medical treatments are bewildering in their variety and inconsistency. Just as people have tried the most outlandish substances on wounds, they have come up with an astonishing number of different systems for treating illness in general, all intended to promote healing. Not uncommonly, these systems are incompatible with one another both in theory and method. Sometimes the methods of one system are expressly prohibited by the rules of another. Yet all have their devoted adherents, and all claim success.

When treatment works and healing ensues, the reason for success may be far from obvious. I want to know why treatments succeed or fail.

IV

A BEWILDERING ARRAY
OF THERAPEUTIC CHOICES

8

Allopathic Medicine I:
Physicians and Surgeons

ALLOPATHIC MEDICINE, the system named disparagingly by Samuel Hahnemann, is now the dominant system of therapeutics in the world. If it cannot claim more practitioners and patients than all other forms of treatment, that is simply because, outside of cities and in nonindustrialized nations, millions of people still rely on herbalists, shamans, priests, and "unorthodox" healers of one sort or another. In Western, urban society allopathy is the only form of medicine taken seriously. Backed by vast sums of money and the intellectual prestige of great universities, decked in all the trappings of modern laboratory science, and supported by an impressive record of clinical success, allopathic medicine exerts an influence on our lives and thinking equal to that of law and religion. So dominant is it that many of its adherents are surprised to learn that other systems of treatment even exist.

Today conventional medicine is under attack. Significant numbers of patients emerge from encounters with it feeling more anger and resentment than gratitude. Alternative practitioners, chafing under its relentless attempts to suppress competition, never miss a chance to portray medical doctors as causers of illness, who cut and poison those seeking help. The holistic medical movement of recent years spends as much time running down allopathic practice as it does building up sensible methods of its own.

Some of the criticisms are unjustified. The slogan that allopaths just treat symptoms seems to me silly. After all, symptoms are what make patients seek medical help, and if treatment does not relieve them, it is a failure in patients' eyes. Good medicine should address underlying causes, too, but treating symptoms is perfectly legitimate, and alternative therapies are not always effective. Putting a person with an itching rash on fruit juice fasts, vitamin supplements, and a program of meditation to improve body-mind harmony will probably not cause harm, but if the itching continues, those actions are off the mark.

Nor is it true that allopaths always make sick people sicker. Regular medicine is the most effective system I know for dealing with many common and serious problems, among them acute trauma; acute infections associated with bacteria, protozoa, some fungi, some parasites, and a few other organisms; acute medical emergencies; and acute surgical emergencies. If I were a victim of a major automobile accident, I would want to be taken to a modern hospital emergency room, not to a homeopath, shaman, herbalist, or chiropractor. If I had overwhelming pneumococcal pneumonia (a bacterial infection of the lungs) I would want to be treated with penicillin. If I contracted intestinal parasites, such as roundworms or amebas, I would take specific allopathic drugs that readily eliminate those creatures without causing much toxicity.

By "acute medical emergencies" I mean such calamities as myocardial infarction (heart attack) and pulmonary edema (accumulation of fluid in the lungs). Allopathic intervention in these conditions often saves lives and reduces the severity and duration of illness. By "acute surgical emergencies" I mean twisted bowels, obstructed bile ducts, inflamed appendices about to burst, hemorrhages in the skull that compress the brain, and the like. In such conditions, prompt and skillful surgery is lifesaving. Regular medicine is also very effective at preventing a number of infectious illnesses by means of immunization and by attention to public health.

Nor is it true that allopathic doctors are all cynical fortune hunters. I know some who are genuine healers and many who come close to the ideal of the hard-working altruist portrayed in old-fashioned novels and movies about doctors.

At the same time, I feel that other criticisms of the system are justified. Scientific (or regular, or orthodox, or conventional, or allopathic) medicine has taken credit it does not deserve for some advances in health. Most people believe that victory over the major infectious diseases of the last century came with the invention of immunizations. In fact, cholera, typhoid fever, tetanus, diphtheria, whooping cough, and the others were in decline before vaccines for them became available — the result of better methods of sanitation, sewage disposal, and distribution of food and water.[1]

The common complaints that medicine today is too expensive, too dangerous, and not effective at treating diseases that really matter are all valid. The expense and risks of the system are direct consequences of its increasing reliance on invasive procedures, technological gadgetry, and dangerous drugs. Its ineffectiveness in certain areas has more to do with theoretical deficiencies. This ineffectiveness is not trivial. Regular medicine is on very shaky ground in attempting to treat such problems as acute infections associated with viruses, nutritional and metabolic diseases, chronic degenerative diseases, allergies and autoimmune diseases, cancer, "psychosomatic disease," and mental illness.

I would look elsewhere than conventional medicine for help if I contracted a severe viral disease like hepatitis or polio, or a metabolic disease like diabetes. I would not seek allopathic treatment for cancer, except for a few varieties, or for such chronic ailments as arthritis, asthma, hypertension (high blood pressure), multiple sclerosis, or for many other chronic diseases of the digestive, circulatory, musculoskeletal, and nervous systems. Although allopaths give lip service to the concept of preventive medicine, for practical purposes they are unable to prevent most of the diseases that disable and kill people today.

It is also true that regular doctors tend to pay attention only to physical bodies, ignoring the mental and spiritual aspects of human beings that are always involved in health and illness. (Indeed, this is the chief theoretical defect of the system.) Furthermore, allopathy as an organized enterprise is not only close-minded toward alternative practices but has waged constant and often unfair wars against other therapeutic systems, regarding them as competition rather than intellectual challenges.

The reader must remember that I am an allopath by education, training, and licensure. I know the system from studying it in medical school, clinics, and doctors' offices, and I know it from experiencing it as a patient. My parents relied on it when I was a child, and I relied on it for much of my life. What I am about to say is based on impressions and experiences gained as both doctor and patient.

In some of the states where I hold medical licenses, the documents state that I am authorized to practice "medicine and surgery." These are the two broad divisions of allopathy, and the boundary between them is of great significance in day-to-day practice, though many patients and laypersons are unaware of it. As a subdivision of allopathic Medicine (with a capital "M"), medicine (with a small "m") embraces such specialties as cardiology, dermatology, gastroenterology, internal medicine, neurology, and psychiatry. The chief surgical specialties are orthopedics, obstetrics and gynecology, urology, thoracic surgery, plastic surgery, neurosurgery, and so forth. Segregation of patients into medical and surgical cases goes on in every allopathic hospital. Although these two forms of practice exist under the same roofs, they constitute very different worlds, often with little communication between them. Surgeons practice surgery; physicians practice medicine. They are distinct breeds of doctor, evolved from different historical antecedents, with different styles and philosophies, as well as different methods. Despite the appearance of the word *surgery* on some of my licenses, I am a physician by inclination and training; I find it easier to discuss surgery because I view it as an outsider.

Today's surgeons evolved from the barber-surgeons of medieval Europe, while physicians of that period came from the elite corps of university students and considered themselves a higher class of practitioners. Of course, surgery really goes back to the earliest attempts to deal with serious wounds, for the defining characteristic of surgery is manipulation of the body, especially its insides, with hands or instruments. The word *surgery* comes originally from a Greek word meaning "working by hand," and ancient Greek doctors relied heavily on surgical techniques. The distinction between physicians and surgeons did not exist in ancient times; it goes back only to the Middle Ages.

Strict criteria exist today for deciding whether a problem is medical or surgical. Nevertheless, I have seen bitter jurisdictional fights over particular hospitalized patients, as well as frequent attempts of one service to unload unwanted cases on the other. For example, acute chest pain is a problem for physicians, whereas acute abdominal pain goes to the surgeons. Occasionally, a patient will arrive at an emergency room complaining of severe and sudden pain around the level of the diaphragm with no obvious diagnosis. If the admitting doctor is on the surgical staff and does not want more work, he may try to dump the case by encouraging the patient to say it hurts worse above the diaphragm. A doctor from the medical staff might do the opposite. When physicians and surgeons get their hackles up at each other, their insults are predictable. Surgeons put down physicians as intellectual nit-pickers, hesitant to take decisive, bold action, while physicians look down at surgeons as unrefined and boorish, ready to cut and mutilate at the slightest excuse.

At its best, modern surgery is a noble skill and craft that sometimes approaches true art. It can dramatically rescue victims of bodily disasters from certain death, as in repairing wounds to vital organs; removing life-threatening tumors, obstructions, and gangrenous limbs; saving babies that cannot be born vaginally; and so on. Surgery may be able to restore function to parts of the body damaged by disease, injury, or accident of birth, can replace some organs on the point of failing (notably kidneys), and, as a cosmetic technique, can genuinely help people whose appearance has been distorted by injury, illness, or aging. When surgery is effective in such cases, it cannot be faulted. I have the highest regard for masters of the craft who know when and when not to use it and who do not hesitate to cut the body when cutting is necessary.

My complaints about surgery go to several areas of abuse and failure: it is often performed unnecessarily and carried out to drastic extremes; its techniques are sometimes worthless; its practitioners are often ignorant of basic principles of health and illness; and its latest practices encourage people to shirk responsibility for maintaining health and preventing serious disease.

Unnecessary surgery is commonplace today, as it probably always has been since the invention of anesthesia and sterile technique. Eager surgeons have removed countless gall bladders, appendices, tonsils, wombs, and teeth that should have been left in place, sometimes in the honest belief that the operations were indicated, sometimes as a crass way of upping their incomes. Done honestly or dishonestly, such injury is an insult to the human body. At best it does patients no good; at worst it does them active harm.

Which organs are targeted for mass removal is a matter of fashion. When I was a youngster in Philadelphia in the mid-1940s, it was rare for a boy or girl to make it through grade school with tonsils and adenoids. Most of us lost them to enthusiastic surgeons who convinced our parents that any recurrent episodes of tonsillitis made tonsillectomy a must. (Of course, physicians abetted this practice by spreading the same falsehood and making the referrals to their colleagues with the scalpels.) We now know that tonsils and adenoids are important organs of the body's immune system. They build lifelong defenses against germs that can make trouble in the respiratory tract and should not be surrendered without very good reason. Nor should a woman be relieved of her uterus because of a history of minor gynecological problems, or anyone of his or her gall bladder because of simple attacks of gall bladder pain.

Never let a surgeon take out a "functionless" organ, either, unless it is really diseased. Functionless organs have a way of turning into very useful ones as soon as researchers admit the possibility of function and try to document it. The "useless" pineal gland in the center of the brain turns out to be a master gland of the endocrine system, regulating biorhythms and hormonal cycles. The "vestigial" thymus gland behind the breastbone is now recognized as a major component of the immune system. I suspect the appendix is another valuable part of that system, probably bolstering defenses against potentially harmful germs in the gut. It should certainly not be cut out without a thought just because the abdomen happens to be open for some other procedure.

The medical profession and responsible surgeons now admit publicly to these excesses. A common estimate is that 25 percent of operations are unnecessary. During the five weeks of a doctors' strike in Los Angeles in 1976, the weekly death rate in hospitals dropped below normal for that time of year. Analysts attributed the drop to unnecessary operations that were not performed during the strike. Emergency surgery went on unchanged, but elective surgery stopped altogether. Once the strike ended, and physicians and surgeons resumed full activity, the death rate rose and stayed above normal for several weeks.[2]

Patients recommended for surgery should always get a second (or even third) opinion from an independent doctor before agreeing to go to the operating room. Some medical societies and government agencies even provide names of reputable surgeons who will give second opinions to patients requesting them.

Surgery that is too extensive is as destructive as surgery that is unnecessary. Radical mastectomy, a horribly mutilating procedure that leaves severe psychological as well as physical scars, is no more effective at preventing recurrences of breast cancer than simple "lumpectomy" or simple mastectomy followed by radiation and other supportive treatment.[3] Despite this fact, surgeons who believe in cutting drastically have been reluctant to abandon the radical mastectomy or listen to the good arguments against it.

Surgeons have often embraced completely worthless operations because they failed to test the procedures experimentally. Their natural inclination to find surgical treatments for more diseases leads them to propose new operations all the time. Because new operations mean more work and higher income, they sometimes become popular before evidence is sought for their value or lack of it.

Angina pectoris had always been a medical problem until surgeons came up with operations to relieve it. One procedure that became fashionable in the 1950s was to open the chest and tie off the internal mammary artery, an artery supplying muscles of the inner chest wall. A branch of this vessel brings blood to the pericardium, the sac enclosing the heart. In theory, tying off the artery below this branch might increase blood flow to an ischemic heart. (The chest wall muscles can find alternative supplies.) Many patients reported disappearance or decrease of anginal pain on recovering from this traumatic operation.

As I explained in chapter 3, angina is notoriously responsive to placebo treatment. Might these patients have improved just because they underwent dramatic surgery? The ethics of controlled studies in this area are sticky, but eventually, a few surgeons put the procedure to a test by performing sham operations on some patients. The patients were told they were undergoing internal mammary artery ligation to bring new blood to their hearts, but, in fact, when their chests were opened, the artery was not tied off. The success rate of sham surgery in alleviating the symptoms of angina was equal to that of the real procedure, proving that this widely endorsed operation acted as a placebo treatment.[4]

Undaunted, the surgeons next came up with a more elaborate procedure: internal mammary artery implant. They now cut the artery and inserted the cut end into a hole poked into the heart muscle, hoping it would sprout new branches to supplement the coronary arteries. Again, patients reported decreases in anginal pain. No one put this procedure to the test of comparison with sham surgery, but, since autopsy data later showed that the implanted arteries did not establish any new blood supplies in heart muscle, any success must also have been a placebo response.

Alleviation of anginal pain by placebos may be perfectly appropriate in some patients if the methods are innocuous, but there is no justification for placebo treatments that expose the body to the trauma and risks of chest surgery. It might be wise to avoid all new and fashionable surgical procedures until they prove their worth over time.

I have met more surgeons than physicians who lack a sense of the basic principles of health and illness, and I find surgeons, as a group, guiltier than physicians of taking up harmful methods based on wrong conceptions. Once, as an intern visiting the surgical ward of a respected hospital, I was shocked to discover that every postoperative patient was receiving intravenous chloramphenicol (Chloromycetin), a powerful and dangerous antibiotic. What could possibly be the reason? When I asked the chief surgical resident, he explained that it was a new policy based on research showing chloramphenicol to be effective at preventing postoperative fever.

It is not wise to give antibiotics to prevent problems; they are better used to treat problems once they arise. It is not wise to overuse antibiotics for anything, because they lose their power when we overuse them. It is not wise to dispense chloramphenicol to all comers, because it is a toxic drug. It is not wise to try to prevent postoperative fever in the first place, or even to treat it unless it gets unusually high and a specific infection can be documented. Fever is often a manifestation of healing, and interfering with it can make it harder for the body to fight invading germs. This kind of practice is a product, I think, of the unsophistication of some surgeons about general matters of health, illness, and treatment. Poor communication between medical and surgical practitioners is one factor in its persistence.

Finally, many of the newer, more drastic surgical procedures, even when they are proved effective, seem to me to do harm by encouraging dangerous ways of thinking about health. The current surgical treatment for angina and coronary artery disease is the coronary bypass, a much publicized and very costly operation that does bring more blood to a diseased heart. The method is to graft sections of veins into the coronary arteries to bypass obstructions. Some patients, incapacitated by heart pain on exertion, are able to resume almost normal activity as soon as they recover from the operation, although their risk of further progression of arterial disease and of death from heart attack may not change.

My uneasiness with this sort of surgery is that it undermines motivation to prevent serious disease in the first place. Most coronary patients have long histories of eating unwisely, getting insufficient exercise, keeping up harmful mental and physical habits (like feeling rage when frustrated, or smoking cigarettes despite signs of arterial disease), and blindly submitting to more and more treatment of symptoms instead of trying to understand and correct unhealthy trends. Availability of coronary bypass surgery, heart transplants, and other seemingly miraculous surgical procedures supports the false idea that we need not bother about preventive maintenance of our bodies or even think about our hearts and other vital organs, because surgeons will be there to rescue us from the results of our folly. As a strong advocate of personal responsibility for maintaining health and managing illness before it becomes too severe to treat by simple methods, I deplore the prevalence of this way of thinking and the role of surgery in fostering it.

Consider these excerpts from an interview with Dr. Denton Cooley of Houston, Texas, the man who pioneered heart transplants in the United States:[5]

> Q: Some say you should be emphasizing prevention instead of such drastic surgery. These operations attract attention and detract from preventive efforts.
> A: Well, nobody has shown how to prevent it. It all sounds good, but from a practical standpoint, it has not paid off . . . I think arteriosclerosis is hereditary. It's a sign of the degenerative process . . . I believe that 85 percent of our destiny in terms of arteriosclerosis is determined at the time of conception. And if you want to spend an ungodly amount of time grappling with the other 15 percent, well, that's your prerogative.

Physicians, who mostly diagnose and treat disease without cutting into the body, like to trace their lineage back to Hippocrates, the great Greek doctor who lived from c. 460 to c. 370 B.C. and practiced and taught on the island of Cos. The system he advocated included both medical and surgical techniques, because all Greek doctors used both. Hippocratic medicine was a rich mixture of wisdom and foolishness.

The teachings of the school at Cos have come down to us in the form of a large collection of writings of very uneven quality. They appear to be the work of many different authors, writing at different times. Perhaps the best of them are from the pen of the master himself, for some of the passages are landmarks in the evolution of medical thought, still relevant to our modern world.

One of the most important Hippocratic ideas was that diseases were products of natural, not supernatural, forces — of sudden changes in weather or diet, for instance, rather than the wrath of demons and capricious gods. Hippocrates also taught that health was the expression of a harmonious balance among internal and external forces, involving mind as well as body, and he clearly stressed the *medicatrix vis naturae*, the healing power of nature: "Nature [*phusis*] heals disease," he wrote. "Inherent mechanisms act automatically as reflexes, much as the reflexes we use in winking the eyelids or moving the tongue, for nature is active without training and without schooling in these essentials."[6]

Hippocrates was the father of environmental medicine, a specialty that has come into its own only in the twentieth century. In the famous treatise "Airs, Waters, and Places," there is a detailed attempt to relate human biology to geography, climate, season, weather, and diet. This treatise was required reading in European and American medical schools until the late 1800s, when modern theories of the specific causation of illness — such as the germ theory — made it seem obsolete.[7]

In practice, Hippocratic doctors made diagnoses on the basis of careful questioning and observation of patients. They selected treatments in a logical and methodical manner, always trying to follow the master's injunction: first, do no harm. When they did, in fact, harm, their folly was the result of ignorance and wrong thinking about the body. They thought infection came from stagnation of blood and so favored bleeding as a treatment, even in cases of severe hemorrhage. Foul, colored pus was an obvious bad sign in a wound, but white, odorless pus was thought to be good and worth encouraging. Hippocratic wound treatments (such as heavy dressings of greasy wool) probably encouraged infection. The Cos school also emphasized purgings and produced them with such dangerous plants as black hellebore (Christmas rose, *Helleborus niger*), a highly irritating, potentially lethal drug. As prisoners of a conceptual scheme based on rigid classification of diseases, foods, drugs, and times of year into categories of hot and cold, moist and dry, Hippocratic doctors recommended regimens in a mechanical way, and some of these must have hindered healing. Their dietary beliefs were quite unsound, for example, since they found fault with almost every vegetable and fruit, often prescribing diets of nothing but meat and cereals.[8]

The best-known legacy from the island of Cos is the Hippocratic oath, still recited by medical students upon receiving their M.D. degrees. It, too, is a mixture of the best and worst of medicine. On the one hand, it enjoins doctors not to harm, not to end life, not to perform abortions, not to molest patients sexually, and to maintain professional confidences. On the other hand, it orders them to keep medical knowledge secret, revealing it only to sons of doctors or others specially admitted to the guild. To this day, a great many physicians engage more in mystification than in education, with the result that the average patient thinks health and illness are such complicated subjects that no one but a doctor can understand or influence them.

Allopathic medicine today contains elements of many post-Hippocratic traditions. It derives from the Roman teachings of Galen, from Arabic medicine (which flowered in the ninth and tenth centuries and entered European practice through Moorish Spain), from the work of medieval alchemist-scientists like Paracelsus, from the academic tradition of great European universities (which culminated in the Age of Heroic Medicine), and, finally, from the new scientific practice that arose in Europe and America in the late 1800s.

Diagnosis in scientific medicine (the word means "to discern" in Greek) is based on the patient's history and physical examination and on laboratory testing. Histories go way back to Hippocrates, and good physicians know the art of taking them well. More than one skillful physician has said that if one asks the right questions, the patient will make the diagnosis for you in his or her own words. Physical examination is also an old technique, but in the last century the use of instruments has changed its nature. Laboratory testing is a purely modern addition. As allopathic doctors have made greater use of technological hardware, diagnosis has become more elaborate, more invasive, more expensive, and more productive of harm.

The use of diagnostic instrumentation dates back to 1819, when a French physician, René Laënnec (1781–1826), introduced the stethoscope. However, the real explosion of diagnostic technology began in the late 1800s with the rapid appearance of four types of procedures and inventions: (1) instruments for or means of visualizing gross anatomical structures, including the ophthalmoscope, laryngoscope, and X-ray; (2) medical use of the microscope to correlate specific diseases with specific germs and tissue changes; (3) devices for measuring body functions in graphical or numerical form, such as the spirometer, sphygmomanometer, and electrocardiogram; and (4) chemical tests of body fluids and tissues.

Doctors have relied on these instruments and procedures more and more in recent years, especially on laboratory tests. In 1954, the Yale–New Haven Hospital performed forty-eight thousand laboratory procedures; in 1959, ninety-eight thousand; and in 1964, two hundred thousand, while the patient census increased only slightly in the same period. In the United States as a whole, about 2 billion laboratory diagnostic tests were done in 1971, 3 billion in 1974, and 4.5 billion in 1976.[9] The upward trend continues. More and more of these tests are now "routine," often lumped together in batches, such as the "liver profile," that doctors can order without much thought.

Some critics call this kind of testing "defensive medicine," because its intent seems more to protect the doctor than to help the patient. As malpractice litigation has increased, doctors have tended to worry more about "covering themselves" and to see extensive diagnostic testing as one means of doing so. Some of them also imagine that numerical test results relieve them of responsibility in identifying medical problems and selecting treatments.

The best diagnosticians I know are all highly trained observers who also have learned to rely on their intuition. They may use laboratory data to supplement their observations and may think they are proceeding scientifically, but, really, they are masters of the ancient art of intuitive diagnosis, for art it is and not science. One old clinician I saw in Boston could "guess" the blood pressure of most patients in the hospital, just by watching them lying in their beds. His guesses were usually right to within a few points. He could not explain how he did it; he just "knew," but his observing was meticulous, including such subtleties as slight motions of the bed as the patient breathed and any visible pulsations of arteries, however slight.

Urinalysis, simple X-rays, and standard blood tests may clinch an intuited diagnosis or provide useful clues to prompt one. Usually, they do not cause much discomfort or damage. Newer tests are another matter, and I see several distinct problems with overuse of them. First, they are directly productive of illness — of *iatrogenic* illness, that is, doctor-caused (from *iatros*, the doctor of ancient Greece). Sampling pieces of liver, lung, and kidney, injecting radiopaque dyes into arteries, exposing patients to great numbers of diagnostic X-rays, injecting powerful drugs for diagnosis rather than treatment are procedures that injure, even kill, certain percentages of patients.

It is ironic that the main argument used by organized allopathy against rival systems like chiropractic concerns their harmfulness. The American Medical Association loves to accuse chiropractors of causing strokes and paralyses by their method of spinal manipulation. No doubt, a few such mishaps have occurred in the hundred years that chiropractors have been cracking necks and backs. Surely, however, the AMA's accusation is a classic case of people in glass houses throwing stones. Compared to such procedures as pneumoencephalography (injecting air into the ventricles of the brain for diagnostic X-rays), angiography (putting catheters and dyes into major arteries), and many other techniques used in every allopathic hospital today, just for diagnosis, the treatment methods of chiropractic and other unorthodox systems are quite harmless.

Aside from the expense and risk they carry, these elaborate procedures discourage physicians from cultivating their own powers of observation and intuition; instead, they encourage belief in a chimerical ideal of diagnosis-by-machine, in which doctors would not exercise their minds at all, just feed the results of laboratory tests into computers and let the computers select the right treatments.*

Another pitfall of allopathic diagnostic method is that doctors often end up treating abnormalities in test results rather than people. This possibility is very real, especially since abnormalities will usually turn up if enough tests are done. In the absence of a sound diagnosis, the patient with a vague problem is likely to be tested till something looks wrong on paper, then be given treatment to correct the test results. Worst of all, the treatment might produce ill effects of its own, creating a further need for intervention and involving the hapless patient ever more deeply with the world of hospitals, clinics, laboratories, and pharmacies.

Of course, the newer diagnostic procedures have their place. Again, the problem is excess — excessive use of them to begin

*It is worth noting that a significant fraction of test results may be in error, due to carelessness in collecting, preserving, transporting, and manipulating specimens.

with and excessive reliance on them in place of simpler methods that are safer, cheaper, and equally helpful when combined with intelligence and experience. Unfortunately, the technological mania that now dominates hospital medicine and medical education makes many people think the older methods of diagnosis are less scientific and therefore less desirable.

9

Allopathic Medicine II: Materia Medica

ONCE A DIAGNOSIS is made, allopathic medical treatment is based almost exclusively on the administration of drugs. So universal is this practice that a patient who does not receive a prescription in the course of a visit to a physician is likely to be disappointed.

The word *physician* stems from the Greek word *phusis*, meaning "nature" and referring to natural medicine and science. (It also gives us *physics*.) Physicians used to be known as "doctors of physic," equivalent to our "doctors of medicine," but their relentless dispensing of drugs gave *physic* a new meaning. It came to denote any drug and specifically one that caused intestinal purging. In the same way, *medicine* has become a synonym for any pharmaceutical product. Physicians today are hard-core materialists. They deal in materia medica, the materials used to treat disease, that is, drugs.

Many allopathic patients are surprised to learn of the existence of wholly drugless systems of treatment. In fact, there are many of them, some now flourishing. Osteopathy started out as such a system, then changed. Chiropractic and acupuncture are persistent examples.

Because I have made a special study of drugs in the course of my professional career, I have a lot to say about them.

Pharmacology is the science of drugs. That word also comes from Greek, derived from an ancient term for poison. The first point I must emphasize is that the only difference between a drug and a poison is dose. All drugs become poisons in high enough doses, and many poisons become useful drugs in low enough doses.* Toxicity (poisoning) from drugs is their great drawback, and allopathic medicine now produces a tremendous amount of it. Adverse drug reactions account for the lion's share of iatrogenic illness — so common that any dedicated patient is sure to experience one sooner or later. They can be as mild as nausea, hives, and drowsiness or as serious as permanent damage to organs and death.

Drug toxicity can be avoided altogether by excluding drugs as a modality of treatment (as in chiropractic) or by diluting them to infinitesimal concentrations (as in homeopathy). Having seen the value of drugs as an allopathic physician, I am inclined to use them when they are clearly indicated. They produce rapid, often immediate results, not only by their direct actions on the body but also indirectly by effectively mobilizing placebo responses. I also feel that doctors should use good judgment about what kinds of drugs they use and how they administer them, in order to reduce the incidence and severity of adverse reactions. Here is the major practical failing of modern allopathic treatment: the kinds of drugs it favors and the ways it puts them into people are very dangerous.

Most of the drugs in current allopathic use come from plants or are synthetic variants of compounds found originally in plants. If we include the antibiotics obtained from molds in this category, the number of plant-derived drugs in the modern materia medica accounts for about 60 or 70 percent of the total.

Until the 1800s most drugs were given by mouth as preparations of crude plants: ground-up leaves, flowers, and roots, or teas, extracts, and tinctures of them. Medicine and botany were then closely allied. Men who studied medicine in universities learned botany. (Only men were admitted to the academies.) At the same time, unschooled herbalists also treated the sick, especially in rural areas, and many of these practitioners were women.

There was much wrong with drug treatment before 1800. Doctors and patients had no assurance that remedies represented to contain particular plants actually contained them. Doses

*Strychnine is an example. Tiny amounts of it are sometimes prescribed to geriatric patients as a cerebral stimulant.

were not standardized. No body of experimental evidence existed on which to base selection of drugs. A great deal of herbalism was — and is — nothing more than superstition crystallized into habit by years of repetition.

A single event in 1803 signaled the end of all this inexactness, one of the early milestones in the development of scientific medicine. In that year a young German pharmacist isolated morphine from opium, for the first time obtaining a pure active principle from a crude vegetable drug. Significantly, he worked first on a psychoactive drug. Drugs that alter mood, perception, and thought have always occupied places of supreme importance in allopathic medicine because they actually make patients feel different (and often better, at least temporarily). Even if they do not improve underlying conditions of disease, they usually make patients go away satisfied. Opium was a most valuable remedy to physicians of the recent past, just as diazepam (Valium) has been to physicians of our era.

Availability of morphine in pure form created a new vision for physicians: the possibility of giving exact doses of known drugs with known effects. Motivated by this vision, chemists and pharmacologists, first in Germany, then in other European countries and America, spent much of the middle nineteenth century methodically studying the plant kingdom in order to discover, isolate, and make available in pure form the active principles of healing plants. By 1870 they had extracted caffeine from coffee, nicotine from tobacco, quinine from cinchona, cocaine from coca, and an array of other pharmacologically active compounds from most of the major medicinal plants.

This work was valuable and important, both theoretically and practically. It revolutionized medical therapeutics and did indeed put an end to the superstition and uncertainty of herbal treatments. It also created new problems of its own.

In their enthusiasm at isolating the active principles of drug plants, researchers of the last century made a serious mistake. They came to believe that all of a plant's desirable properties could be accounted for by a single compound, that it would always be better to conduct research and treat disease with the purified compound than with the whole plant. In this belief, they forgot the plants once they had the active principles out of them, called all the other principles "inactive," and advanced the notion that prescribing refined white powders was more scientific and up to date than using crude green plants.

The idea that plants owe their effects to single compounds is simply untrue.[1] Drug plants are always complex mixtures of chemicals, all of which contribute to the effect of the whole. It is true that one compound will often be present in the greatest amount and will often reproduce the most interesting activity of the plant. For example, opium contains twenty-two different drugs. There is more morphine than any of the others, and morphine is certainly responsible for most of the euphoria and analgesia produced by opium. It is fair to say that morphine is the dominant constituent of opium, but not that it is the sole active principle. Codeine is also active, as are papaverine and all the others. Give some patients opium and some morphine, and you will see qualitative differences in response. Morphine is not just opium in a more concentrated and convenient form.

The erroneous idea that plants and isolated active principles are equivalent has become fixed dogma in pharmacology and medicine today. As a physician with a background in botany who has studied the effects of medicinal plants, I find it difficult to explain to my colleagues that coffee is not caffeine, coca is not cocaine, and other purified drugs are not the same as the plants they come from. The trouble is that few, if any, pharmacologists and physicians now have firsthand knowledge of the plants. They know only the pure derivatives and the statements repeated in textbooks and lecture halls for the past hundred years equating the two.

It is useful to know how drug plants differ from pure compounds derived from them, because the differences have great practical import.

In general, isolated and refined drugs are much more toxic than their botanical sources. They also tend to produce effects of more rapid onset, greater intensity, and shorter duration. Sometimes they fail to reproduce desirable actions of plants they come from, and sometimes they lack natural safeguards present in those plants. They also lend themselves to methods of administration favoring abuse and toxicity. There are logical explanations for all of these differences.

A sound principle of pharmacology, one that may seem to go against common sense, is that the intensity of a drug's effect depends more on how fast its concentration in the bloodstream and target organs increases than on how much of it is taken. A large dose of a drug entering the bloodstream slowly will be milder than a small dose entering rapidly. When blood concentrations of drugs rise quickly, their actions are fast, intense, short-lasting, and, often, near or in the range of toxic rather than therapeutic effects.

Crude preparations of medicinal plants taken by mouth release active principles into the bloodstream relatively slowly. The concentrations of these principles are usually low, and often they are bound up with inert components that inhibit quick release into the digestive tract. Refined drugs, especially when converted to water-soluble salts, wind up in the stomach in much higher concentration and diffuse out of it much faster. Moreover, refined drugs may be put into the bloodstream in more direct ways.

The hypodermic syringe was invented in 1853 by a Scottish allopath named Alexander Wood. His wife became the world's first morphine addict. That delicious irony says all one needs to know about the relative risks of oral administration of crude drugs versus intravenous administration of refined ones.

Not only are the active principles of medicinal plants highly diluted and less soluble, they are also combined with other substances that modify their actions. Coca leaves contain about 0.5 percent cocaine along with thirteen other pharmacologically active compounds. Cocaine accounts for about 70 percent of the total of this family of drugs and reproduces the most spectacular effects of the leaves: topical anesthesia, stimulation, and euphoria. Accordingly, scientists of the last century dubbed cocaine the active principle of coca, dismissed the other thirteen compounds as "inactive" (or "secondary" or "minor") without bothering to determine their effects, and stopped studying coca once they had access to pure cocaine. Finally, they released cocaine to the world as a new wonder drug, supposed to embody all the therapeutic virtues attributed to the leaves by countless generations of South American Indians.

The result was disaster, for excessive and careless use of cocaine caused serious, even lethal, toxicity and much dependence. Nor did cocaine bring the considerable medical benefits of coca to the Western world. It did open the era of local anesthesia but that success is offset by widespread and increasing abuse of cocaine, now supplied by black markets. South American Indians use coca leaves but do not abuse them. Our problems stem directly from the decision of scientific medicine to value the refined white powder over the green plant. I do not doubt that one of the reasons coca is more useful and less harmful than cocaine is modification of the activity of that drug by the host of related secondary compounds found within coca naturally.[2]

The possibility that secondary compounds of medicinal plants may be valuable in their own right or may modify the effects of dominant compounds in good ways seems unremarkable to me. Nevertheless, I find I have to explain it to allopathic physicians and pharmacologists with great patience. I notice that I make many of these people uneasy when I impute any "wisdom" to nature; they seem to resent the suggestion that natural substances may be better than manmade ones.

All I can say is that, empirically, I find such a difference, at least in the case of medicinal plants versus isolated drugs. Whenever I have had a chance to observe or experience firsthand treatment with a plant and treatment with a refined derivative of the plant, I have found the latter to be more dangerous and sometimes less useful.

One of the plants I have used in my own practice is Chinese ephedra (*Ephedra sinica*), a leafless shrub of arid regions related to coniferous trees. Chinese ephedra is the oldest medicinal plant of which we have written records. Ancient Chinese doctors knew it as *ma huang* at least five thousand years ago and recommended it for asthma and respiratory congestion. Many species of *Ephedra* grow throughout the world, including several in western North America known as Mormon tea or squaw tea, but the Chinese species is strongest and the only one recognized officially for medical use. This plant is the natural source of the drug ephedrine, a stimulant and relaxant of bronchial smooth muscle, still much used as an allopathic treatment for asthma.

Not all asthmatics respond to ephedrine, but those who do, while admitting its effectiveness in relieving attacks, usually complain about side effects: jitteriness, insomnia, and a feeling of being drained of energy the following day. When I have taught such patients to use Chinese ephedra tea as an alternative, most of them find they can obtain similar relief, though of somewhat slower onset, with none or little of ephedrine's toxicity. I do not know the exact reasons for this difference. Probably, the tea provides ephedrine in a dilute form, possibly modified by secondary compounds, without causing sharp spikes in blood concentration of the drug. Whatever the reasons, the difference I report is an observable fact.

Toxicity of drugs is often rated by a number called the therapeutic ratio: the ratio of the minimum dose producing toxic effects to the minimum dose producing desired effects. For many drugs in current allopathic use that number is between 10 and 20. Ten times the dose of aspirin used to relieve a bad headache may cause symptoms of salicylate poisoning, a severe reaction. For some drugs the ratio is much smaller. Digitalis drugs, used to treat failing hearts, have quite small margins of safety, with a therapeutic ratio of about 2.

Digitalis, or foxglove, provides further evidence for the inherent safety of natural drugs. Its value was unknown to European allopaths before 1775 because it was used exclusively by women herbalists, and no university-educated male physician would condescend to talk to any of these "old wives." As a result, physicians were powerless to treat a condition called dropsy, the accumulation of fluid in the lower extremities with swelling of the feet and ankles. Dropsy (or dependent edema, as we call it today) has various causes, the most important being failure of the heart as a pump and consequent building of back pressure in the veins. Heart failure often develops slowly and progresses gradually but persistently, leading to eventual disability and death. Some of England's old wives could cure dropsy with herbal teas.

In 1775 a young English physician named William Withering was persuaded by his fiancée to visit an herbalist in Shropshire who had such a cure. He realized that the key ingredient of the tea she prescribed was foxglove leaves. After trying out similar preparations on his own patients, he wrote a treatise titled "An Account of the Foxglove and Some of Its Medical Uses" that established his fame and brought this valuable plant into the mainstream of Western medicine, where it has ever since remained.

Until the 1920s, the only form of digitalis used in medicine was the whole leaf, usually dried, ground, and encapsulated. In that decade, the active principles of digitalis, having been identified and isolated, became available to doctors in pure form. The first to be used was digitoxin, the second digoxin. Soon these chemicals supplanted use of the leaf. Today, it is unheard of for physicians to treat heart-failure patients with digitalis leaf; they now use digoxin or one of its relatives. It is even difficult to obtain pharmaceutical preparations of digitalis leaf anymore. Hospital pharmacies do not stock them, and few physicians would know how to use them if they could get them.

Digitalis drugs correct irregular heartbeats and may increase the strength of heart contractions. Although they are supremely useful, their safety margin is so narrow and their toxicity so grave that pharmacologists put much emphasis on the importance of recognizing the symptoms of overdose when teaching medical students about these drugs.

When I studied pharmacology in 1965, the manner of this teaching puzzled me. I was taught to watch for three successive stages to digitalis toxicity. The symptoms of the first stage are supposed to be gastrointestinal, usually nausea and vomiting. The second stage is marked by benign, or atrial, arrhythmias of the heart: that is, the upper chambers of the heart begin to beat in abnormal rhythms. (Since the atria contribute little to the pumping mechanics of the heart as a whole, these disturbances are not very serious.) The third stage is ventricular arrhythmia, in which the main or lower chambers of the heart beat irregularly; this condition can be fatal within a few minutes. Obviously, one must identify symptoms of digitalis overdosage early and correct them before the third stage occurs.

But after this description, I was told never to expect to see the first stage, never to expect gastrointestinal symptoms. I could not understand the logic of creating three stages to something if one of them never happens. In fact, in my medical training I never did see anybody complain of nausea or vomiting when they were overdosed with digitalis drugs. I only saw people go into atrial arrhythmias that were often first noticed on electro-cardiogram, and I saw many such cases.

I asked my instructors why they taught the subject in that way, but they could not give me a good answer. All they could say was, "That's the way it is," or "That's what all the books say," or "That's how we were taught." It took me a long time to find a good answer. When I did, it made perfect sense.

Some years after graduating from medical school, I was talk-ing with an old physician about my belief in the relative safety of plant forms of drugs. He said, "I'll give you an example of that. Long ago, I always treated my heart-failure cases with dig-italis leaf. They always got sick to their stomachs if you gave them too much. They never got heart irregularities, and you could cut the dose back at leisure. You could have them come in once a week for increasing doses and for checks on heart function, until one week they might say, 'I don't know what's wrong with me; I can't keep any food down; I feel terrible.' Then you could cut the dose. They were never near the point of an arrhythmia. When digitoxin and digoxin came in, I switched to using them, like everyone else. Now patients who get too much don't get sick to their stomachs. They develop irregular heart-beats right off. I haven't used digitalis leaf in years and don't know anyone who has. I'm not sure I could even still get it."

Clearly, here is the origin of the mysterious teaching about three stages of digitalis toxicity. It dates from a time when only the leaf was used, and the elusive first stage is a characteristic of the leaf, not of its purified derivatives. I have since interviewed other older practitioners, all of whom confirm this idea.

Whatever the compounds are in foxglove that irritate the stomach, they are not digoxin and digitoxin. They are not the heart-stimulating compounds at all but, rather, associate com-pounds that occur along with them, a suggestion supported by at least one study in the scientific literature.[3] In other words, the whole plant has certain built-in safety mechanisms that are lost when the cardiotonic elements are refined out and used in pure form. Call this the wisdom of nature if you like, or don't if you don't like; it remains an empirical truth.

Even with these facts in hand, I find it hard to convince al-lopathic physicians of the virtues of digitalis leaf. Many of them just dismiss it as old-fashioned. Some argue that with the leaf you cannot know exactly what dose you are giving. That is true, but the point is that the vastly greater safety margin of whole digitalis makes it unnecessary to be so exact about dose. Besides, standardization of botanical drugs is not impossible. When pharmaceutical companies sold digitalis leaf, they produced capsules of uniform strength by growing and harvesting the plant under constant conditions and by testing the material on animals. It is when you inject digoxin intravenously that you have to be precise to tenths of milligrams to avoid poisoning patients.

Another argument, also valid, is that digitalis leaf acts slowly. Intravenous digoxin may change heart function within minutes, whereas the leaf taken orally may not produce a satisfactory change for two weeks or more. To defend the merits of digitalis leaf is not to say the purified derivatives are worthless. It can be lifesaving to have intravenous digoxin in reserve for cases of sudden heart failure (an occasional complication of myocardial infarction and other heart ailments), because sudden heart failure is a medical emergency that can lead to death within hours if not corrected promptly. In my experience, however, the percentage of such emergencies out of the total cases of heart failure presenting to physicians is small. Usually hearts fail gradually over months and years as cardiac muscle weakens. Many of these patients could be treated successfully with digitalis leaf as outpatients. They and their doctors would enjoy the luxury of a comfortable margin of drug safety, now lost with total reliance on the isolated compounds.

The complete disappearance of digitalis leaf from modern allopathic practice — so complete that the reason for listing three stages of toxicity has been forgotten — is revealing of the attitude of allopaths about drugs. They prefer substances that cause immediate, dramatic changes in patients, even at the expense of much greater risk. The crisis orientation of today's hospitals encourages this inclination and reinforces the belief, now over a century old, that refined white powders make for more scientific therapy than crude botanicals or other dilute forms of medication.

Once pharmaceutical chemists had pure active principles to work with, they began to tinker with those molecules, seeking to improve on them. I see nothing wrong with attempts to improve on nature. Indeed, I think they are a noble human activity. The development of beautiful flowers and delicious fruits and vegetables from much less appealing wild progenitors shows how responsive nature is to human intervention and how welcome can be the products of such effort. Of course, the outcome is determined by wise or foolish selection of natural traits to develop. Selection and breeding to yield hard, uniform tomatoes that are unpleasant to eat but more suitable for mass production and distribution are motivated by greed for money rather than concern for human welfare.

I am afraid that the choices of medical scientists in modifying natural drugs have also mostly been foolish, because they have valued increased potency and pharmacological power and rapid action over safety and overall quality of effect. Some of their creations have been true blessings, many more are mixed blessings, and some have been curses to humanity.

By studying the molecular configuration of cocaine, pharmaceutical chemists were able to synthesize analogs of it that acted as local anesthetics but were less toxic and did not cause general stimulation. These compounds — procaine (Novocain) is an example — are useful, safe drugs that eliminate much of the pain of minor surgery and dentistry and allow safe nerve blocks for more major operations.

Aspirin is a mixed blessing, created first in a German laboratory by tacking an acetic acid group onto salicylic acid, the natural analgesic, anti-inflammatory, and antipyretic (fever-reducing) substance in the bark of some willow trees (and named for the willow genus, *Salix*). Native Americans drank white willow bark tea to relieve aches and pains, and some devotees of herbal treatment still do. When chemists isolated salicylic acid and gave it to doctors to try on patients in pure form, its advantages and disadvantages were obvious. Salicylic acid is faster and more powerful than willow bark tea at relieving pain but also extremely irritating to the stomach. Aspirin has the greater strength of the refined compound with less of its irritating quality. It has proved itself over time as a generally valuable remedy.

Nevertheless, we pay a significant price for totally rejecting willow bark in favor of aspirin. That drug is terribly overused today, with many consumers regarding it as not much stronger than after-dinner mints. Actually, aspirin is a powerful drug, affecting many systems of the body, some in ways not yet understood. It is routinely administered to patients with slight or moderate fevers, when those fevers would better be left as they are. It causes marked irritation of the stomach: even ordinary doses can produce microscopic hemorrhages in the lining of that organ. Finally, it is a major cause of serious poisoning in our society, both accidental and deliberate, in both adults and children.

A very similar chemical change enabled chemists to step up the potency of morphine. By adding two acetic acid groups to it, they created a new opiate made available to the medical profession in 1898 and marketed enthusiastically for a short time as a safe and superior cough suppressant. That drug was heroin, placed under severe restrictions when its potential for abuse and toxicity became clear.

In this century, the creation of new drugs in laboratories has shifted from universities to industry, with large pharmaceutical companies vying with one another to come up with marketable innovations. Greater potency, strength, and rapidity of action remain the qualities sought, and, increasingly, novelty has become a desired characteristic.

I am not much of a fan of the pharmaceutical industry. Many of its products are worthless, destined to be forgotten once their novelty wears off; all of them are grossly overpriced, much of the profit going toward lavish advertising and other forms of salesmanship intended to persuade the allopathic physician to prescribe one company's brands over another's. The list of really worthwhile drugs in the therapeutic repertory is not all that long, and many of them date from before the beginnings of the modern pharmaceutical industry: morphine, digitalis, quinine, and so forth.

I must relate the story of my own experience of working briefly for one major pharmaceutical house. In 1961, after my first year of college, I took a summer job as assistant to a general practitioner in Philadelphia who had a contract with this company to run clinical tests on new drugs. The doctor was a friend of the vice-director of a large state mental hospital and so had free access to patients as test subjects. The hospital made no effort to treat most of the thousands of patients it housed but merely maintained them in minimally adequate conditions. The staff doctors were mostly foreign, some with little command of English. Many patients saw a doctor only once a year and then for just a few minutes.

In those days, the Food and Drug Administration's regulation of new drugs and drug testing was considerably looser than it is now. Manufacturers did not have to prove the efficacy of a new drug in order to market it, just basic safety. Test results were not always scrutinized carefully, and no strict rules existed for the use of patients as guinea pigs.

The drug company of this story had just come up with a "new" tranquilizer, actually a variant of chlorpromazine (Thorazine), the best-selling product of a competitor. The company wanted to figure out how to sell its invention. People who do not know the ways of pharmaceutical companies imagine that they study diseases and try to invent drugs to fill medical needs. Such is not the case. More often, the companies hire chemists specializing in particular classes of molecules, and those chemists try to come up with new patentable molecules. A patentable molecule is one different enough from a molecule some other company already markets to merit a patent of its own. When a company obtains a patent on a molecular variant of an existing drug, the job then is to find a way to sell it. That is, the company attempts to fit a disease to its chemical.

In this case the company owned a molecule like Thorazine, expected it to have effects on psychiatric patients, and wanted to know what it might be good for. They had completed basic animal tests to determine gross toxicity and now had government clearance to start tests on humans. They had no idea at all what conditions it might help; they asked us to pick samples of chronic psychiatric patients, all with different diagnoses, give the patients increasing doses of the new drug, and see what happened.

Because the doctor who had the contract was too busy to do much of the work himself, he let me run the project. (I was passed off to the hospital as a medical student.) Not having done anything of the sort before, I had to figure out most of the procedures for myself. I went into locked wards full of psychotic patients, choosing those to receive the new tranquilizer. I was to use placebos, too, but in single-blind fashion only; that is, I knew who got the real drug, but the patients did not.

I arranged for the drug to be started and increased in dosage each week. I also checked the patients every few days, taking blood pressure and blood samples, trying to talk to them to determine mental status, and so forth. It did not take long to see that the drug had devastating side effects. Most patients on it got dizzy, and many fell over or fainted when they tried to stand up because it unbalanced the postural reflexes that maintain blood pressure in an upright position. One man was injured badly as a result of such a fall, and one woman died of a heart attack, possibly precipitated by a sudden drop in blood pressure on getting out of bed. The drug also caused bed-wetting, which did not endear it to patients or nurses. These effects were not subtle; they were gross and obvious.

After eight weeks, the testing ended, and it fell to me to write up the results for the manufacturer. Lacking experience in preparing such a report and having no model to follow, I just structured it as I thought I should, noting all the effects I observed and documenting them with figures. There were no good effects to report. The doctor I worked for approved what I wrote, and we sent it in.

Some months later, the company wrote back to us. They thanked us for our data and told us the results of other work with the drug. It had been tested in twelve locations around the country. Ten of the reports came back favorable. One was neutral. Ours was the only unfavorable one. The company then said that because ours was the "best documented," they had decided not to market the drug as a new psychiatric medication.

The only reason our report was the best documented must have been my inexperience at writing reports on drug testing. What did that say about the quality of the others? How could ten other investigators fail to notice and report the obvious and alarming side effects?

Here ends part one of this saga. Part two took place eight years later. I was then interning at a hospital in San Francisco and used to receive a great volume of junk mail from pharmaceutical companies. One day I found in my mailbox a promotional announcement from the company I had worked for.

The announcement described a new drug just going on the market. Yes, it was the same one. Only now the company was not pushing it as a remedy for mental disorders but as a pain reliever for nonambulatory patients and as a pre-anesthetic medication to calm patients before surgery. All of the side effects I had noted were listed in fine print under "Warnings," including the possibility of dangerous, even fatal, drops in blood pressure on standing upright. The company had invested in that molecule and had not let go of it. After eight years, they had found a way to sell it, and they continue to sell it to this day.

I do not think this story is atypical of pharmaceutical companies or many of their products. Compounding the problem is widespread ignorance among physicians about the effects and interactions of the drugs they use. When most allopathic doctors want information on drugs, they turn to industry publications like the *Physicians' Desk Reference*,[4] rather than to objective, impartial sources. They are also strongly influenced by advertisements in medical journals and by the efforts of company detail men, specially trained salesmen who visit doctors to persuade them to prescribe particular brands. The techniques of persuasion can be outrageous, gift giving being common. One detail man, who was always welcome at the hospital where I interned, would hand out free bottles of amphetamines in hopes that we would prescribe more of his company's newest and most expensive antibiotic, one not shown to differ significantly from its older relatives except in appearance and cost to the patient.

The average patient in a hopsital today is placed on half a dozen drugs simultaneously. How some of these chemicals react with each other is anybody's guess. Moreover, a significant percentage of drug doses in hospitals involve errors: the wrong drug, the wrong patient, the wrong dose, the wrong time. As I wrote earlier, adverse drug reactions are the leading variety of iatrogenic illness. The kinds of drugs allopaths choose to give favor these reactions. They also account for a high proportion of soaring medical costs, often fail to improve health, and frequently make patients dependent on pharmacies and pills.

Even in the last century, when milder forms of drugs were more in use, Oliver Wendell Holmes commented: "I firmly believe that if the whole materia medica as now used could be sunk to the bottom of the sea, it would be all the better for mankind and all the worse for the fishes."[5] Earlier still, Voltaire penned this magnificent snipe: "Physicians pour drugs of which they know little, to cure diseases of which they know less, into humans of which they know nothing."[6]

The excesses of drugging in allopathic medicine are one of its worst sins. Yet those excesses are merely symptoms of conceptual problems at the core of the therapeutic system that dominates our world.

10

Allopathic Medicine III: Sins of Omission

PERMIT ME to reiterate my belief in the value of much of regular medicine and its superiority over all rival systems in treating the problems I listed at the beginning of chapter 8. I have seen allopaths save many lives. I have also experienced cures of illness in myself after allopathic treatment.

Once, at the end of a stay with a tribe of Amazonian Indians in Colombia, I scraped a patch of skin from the side of my right hand while stroking a strange musical instrument fashioned from a turtle shell. I washed the raw area in a river, having no medications with me, but within hours it was inflamed and painful, probably infected by some aggressive tropical germs. My low resistance from a period of fatiguing travel in a difficult environment must have favored the infection. I was unable to reach an outpost of Western civilization for 48 hours. By then, the infection had escaped local containment. Red streaks extended up my arm, leading to swollen lymph nodes in the armpit. I was weak and had a fever. I was very glad to be able to start antibiotic therapy in addition to using such simple measures as bed rest, hot soaks, and disinfection with hydrogen peroxide. The combination turned the tide in my favor within a day and a half.

What I have complained of in chapters 8 and 9 are allopathic *excesses*: excessive surgery, excessive use of drugs of excessive potency, and so forth. Antibiotics are wonderful tools to have in reserve for emergencies. Physicians just prescribe them much too often. I would guess they are not really indicated at least 75 percent of the times they are dispensed. Not only is such use unnecessary, it costs money, produces toxicity, and, by selecting resistant germs, decreases the effectiveness of the antibiotics for everyone in the future.

Here I want to focus on *deficiencies* of allopathy, conceptual inadequacies that render it unable to treat many of the most common and serious diseases that plague us.

I find allopathic medicine glaringly deficient in theory and philosophy of any sort.

Sit a homeopath down and ask about the theory of the system, and he or she should have no trouble explaining it. Health for the homeopath is a state of balance reflecting the divine harmony of nature; disease is a state of imbalance characterized by sets of symptoms peculiar to individual patients. Healing comes from within and can be encouraged by administering specially diluted preparations of drugs shown to reproduce those symptom patterns in healthy people.

An articulate chiropractor should be able to give an equally ready and concise response. Health is a state of perfect balance and adjustment of bodily systems, especially of the musculoskeletal and nervous systems. The ultimate cause of disease is maladjustment of spinal vertebrae, causing dysfunction of nerves and blood vessels and thereby of other organs. Treatment is a matter of correcting the maladjustments by means of spinal manipulation, allowing the body to resume normal function.

A Chinese acupuncturist would say something of this sort: health of the body is the microcosmic reflection of the harmony of heaven, representing a state of balance in the complementary and opposing forces of the universe. Disease begins as an imbalance in those forces, producing either excesses or deficiencies of basic life energy in particular organs. If not corrected, these imbalances eventually produce physical changes in the material body. Treatment consists of manipulating energy flow around the body in order to draw excess energy away from organs with too much and redirect it to organs with too little.

I make no judgments here about the validity of these conceptions. I just note their existence as sources of logical unity and power in systems of treatment.

Now try asking an allopath the same question. You will not

get much of an answer. Allopaths may say that health is the absence of disease, but they have no clear conception or theory of what disease is, nor any general concept of treatment. Lacking a clear and unified theory, allopathy is a vast and cumbersome body of data concerning the identification of specific, physical agents of disease and the use of particular treatments directed against those agents.

One consequence of this deficiency in theory is the difficulty of teaching the system. Medical school curriculums are notoriously unwieldy and inefficient because teachers have to expose students to endless facts and details. If they could teach a basic conceptual framework on which to organize the details, medical teaching could be simplified greatly.

Worse, lack of any clear concept of health leads most medical doctors to pay more attention to disease. I heard the word *health* mentioned very infrequently during four years of medical school and one of internship, though I listened to innumerable lectures and seminars on diseases. One incisive commentator, an M.D. and pathologist, has said: "If we measure interest by activities rather than by protestations, physicians have been and are, for the most part, as little interested in health as soldiers in peace."[1] Allopathic doctors give lip service to preventive medicine, but what they mean by that term are mostly superficial matters relating to public sanitation and mass immunization against epidemic diseases. The preventive activities of regular doctors are minimal; mostly they wage war against diseases once they have developed and against agents that transmit them, which they mistakenly see as final causes.

War and battle imagery are abundant in allopathic literature and thinking. The pharmacopeia is the "therapeutic arsenal." New machines for diagnosis and therapy are "new weapons" against disease. Specific drugs are "magic bullets"* to be aimed at pathogenic organisms. I have in my files an arresting pharmaceutical ad for a new antibiotic: twin syringes filled with the liquid lie crossed like dueling pistols in the depressions of a velvet-lined gun case. The American Cancer Society urges us to

*This phrase was popularized by the title of a classic Hollywood medical movie made in 1940, *Dr. Ehrlich's Magic Bullet*, about the inventor of the first specific drug treatment for syphilis.

"fight cancer" with checkups and checks, while the National Cancer Institute tries to reassure an ever more skeptical public that we are "winning the war" on that disease.

Warring against bacteria and other potential agents of disease often increases their harmfulness in the long run, as the appearance of resistant strains of staphylococcus and gonococcus shows. Besides, this way of thinking hardly allows for attention to health and for efforts to define, understand, and maintain it. As a result, the body of the average allopathic patient becomes a perpetual war zone for the testing and use of therapeutic weaponry; the best hope is for occasional cease-fires.

Lack of a coherent philosophy of the abstract notions of health as wholeness, perfection, and balance encourages allopaths to pay attention mostly to the concrete manifestations of illness. The materialism of Western society and science has fostered this tendency to an extreme degree, so that most medical doctors do not admit the importance or even the reality of nonmaterial factors in determining health and illness. Belief, thought, emotion, and spiritual forces are phantoms to allopaths, sometimes mentioned in casual conversation but never accorded scientific relevance. This professional blindness to vital components of human beings keeps many doctors from understanding or making serious use of such phenomena as placebo responses, hypnosis, faith healing, and suggestion. It keeps them from seeing the significance of folk cures for warts, spontaneous remissions of cancer, yogic control of supposedly involuntary functions, and so forth, and from appreciating the body's own capacity for healing. Doctors who ignore the mental and spiritual dimensions of their patients will never be able to teach about health or practice genuine preventive medicine.

It is the materialistic bias of scientific medicine that also leads it to make drugs the universal modality of treatment (except when surgery is indicated), to value very potent refined or synthetic drugs above milder, natural ones, and to embrace technological gadgetry for diagnosis and treatment with greater enthusiasm than simple methods not requiring elaborate equipment.

So it is the conceptual deficiency of the system that produces its sins of commission: the adverse reactions to drugs and diagnostic techniques and the escalating expense. Equally, this deficiency is responsible for allopathy's sins of omission: its failure to practice real preventive medicine and its inability to deal with all the categories of disease where specific, material causes have not been found (such as cancer) or have not been matched to magic bullets (such as viral infections). As I will show in a later section, the power of alternative medicine in moderating some of these problems is explained by its recognition and use of the nonmaterial determinants of health and disease.

Since regular medicine sees itself engaged in a never-ending struggle against illness, it is not surprising that patients are sucked into the same way of thinking and find themselves more and more dependent on the system once they make initial contact with it. I consider this common pattern a serious black mark against allopathy, because I believe interactions with practitioners should make patients more aware of their bodies and how to manage them, more self-reliant and independent of outside help. What I usually see in people who go exclusively to allopaths is a trend to more frequent visits, more medication, reinforcement of the notion that health and illness are beyond the comprehension of ordinary folk, and insidiously progressive dependence on doctors, pharmacies, and hospitals.

Alternative systems are sometimes no better in this regard, of course. Chiropractic, for one, is flagrantly guilty of breeding dependence in patients. Treatment does not have to be that way, however. Patients should be aware of the danger of dependence. If it seems too great, they should consider another form of therapy or, at least, question the recommendations of practitioners rather than accept them blindly.

I could write at much greater length about allopathic medicine, but others have aired their complaints in more detail. I will not spend as much time on other therapeutic systems as I have on allopathy, not because the alternatives are less interesting or less deserving of criticism, but because they influence the lives of most of us less than regular medicine. However, I conclude with four case examples to illustrate the practical problems resulting from allopathy's conceptual limitations.

A young man, a lawyer, aged twenty-six, in generally good health, received a disturbing letter from a leading university hospital, where he was treated as a child. It informed him that sixteen years previously he had been exposed to X-rays directed at his thymus to make it shrink, then a fashionable medical procedure. It went on to say that physicians now were seeing increased incidence of thyroid cancer in the people who underwent this treatment, and it urged him to have thyroid function tests done. He asked me what I thought. I advised him not to worry.

This patient came to me some time ago, and he has remained in good health, though his faith in doctors is not as strong as it once was. When he was irradiated as a child, allopathic physicians were ignorant of the importance of the thymus as a key component of the immune system, especially active in childhood. This organ lies behind the breastbone and shrinks up in adolescence. X-rays make it shrink immediately, and not so long ago, doctors advocated their use as a way of hastening the disappearance of this "functionless" organ. They even invented a new and universal disease, "thymic hypertrophy," to describe the normal thymus of childhood.

I cannot excuse such activity as simple ignorance. It is more an arrogant disregard of the wholeness and holiness of the human body. To label an organ useless because you do not understand it and then to injure or destroy it with a technological weapon is the antithesis of good medicine and concern for health. Only allopaths are guilty of atrocities of this sort. No homeopath, chiropractor, acupuncturist, herbalist, or shaman would ever dream of treating the body in such a fashion.

Another young man, this one also in his midtwenties, came to me recently. He worked as a nurse on the urology ward of a large urban hospital and had developed chronic prostatitis. The prostate gland contributes secretions to semen and is susceptible to chronic, low-grade, bacterial infections that ascend to it from the lower urinary tract and persist in deep recesses poorly supplied with blood. Lack of good blood supply reduces the possibility of healing and makes it hard for antibiotics to reach the site of infection. Frequently, after an initial, acute episode, prostatitis will seem to disappear, only to flare up repeatedly when the gland is stressed or resistance is low. This man had had three recurrences, all of them treated with antibiotics. The last treatment had failed, however, and a urologist in charge of the case, one of the senior doctors of his ward, recommended surgery to remove the gland. The patient wanted a second opinion from me.

I gave him one in strong terms. Prostatectomy in such a young man is totally unjustified. That recommendation seemed to be based on the failure of a course of antibiotic therapy, as if that were the only way to affect prostatic disease. Prostatitis can be treated by a variety of simpler methods: increasing fluid intake and urinary output, drinking cranberry juice as a urinary tract antiseptic, eliminating caffeine from the diet, changing the frequency of ejaculation, avoiding mechanical stresses (like horseback or motorcycle riding), and receiving regular massages of the gland from a finger inserted in the rectum.

Although this patient lived in the desert, and I saw him in the hot part of the year, no doctor had told him of the importance of drinking a lot of water (dehydration renders the prostate more susceptible to infection) or of avoiding caffeine (and especially coffee, which irritates the entire urogenital tract in many people and certainly aggravates an inflamed prostate) or of the usefulness of prostatic massage. His condition subsided when he applied these measures conscientiously.

The readiness of an allopathic doctor to go right to the most extreme, expensive, and risky methods without even thinking of simple, safe, and cheap ones is, I am afraid, typical of practice today. It demonstrates profound lack of faith in the body's innate healing abilities. Of course, drastic treatments are sometimes required, but I fear that very many patients have suffered them needlessly only because they did not question the advice of doctors and explore alternative methods.

The third case concerns a personal experience. In 1959 I set out on a long series of travels through Asia, the Middle East, and Europe. My family doctor gave me all the recommended immunizations, along with a supply of a drug to treat the intestinal disturbances I was likely to suffer. The drug was an iodine compound called iodochlorhydroxyquin, sold under the brand name Entero-Vioform. It was very popular then and for years thereafter, widely prescribed to travelers and generally considered an effective remedy for the routine diarrheas of travelers — those common and uncomfortable maladies known as "turista" in Latin America, "Delhi belly" in India, and a variety of other colorful names.

I took my Entero-Vioform faithfully from Hong Kong through Egypt, whenever my intestines acted up too badly. They were never right in any of that part of the world. Only when I reached Istanbul did they quiet down. Then they mostly functioned normally as I made my way west.

What I had experienced was a syndrome I now call the "displaced bowel," and I am still surprised that so few allopathic doctors and patients understand it.

Our intestines work in intimate relationships with the bacteria in our environment. There are staggering numbers of germs in all the food we eat and water we drink. Far from causing trouble, these organisms live in balance with our intestinal cells, enabling them to digest food. Animals raised from birth in germ-free environments have abnormal intestines that neither look nor work right.

Germs differ from place to place, just as geography, plant life, and people differ. When we travel to other countries — especially those where food, people, and customs are very different from our own — our intestines are suddenly faced with unfamiliar bacteria. They must learn to adapt to them and strike a new balance in order to keep functioning harmoniously. Until they achieve that balance, they suffer the displacement syndrome. They cannot digest food properly; some of it putrifies, resulting in irritating breakdown products responsible for much of the pain and diarrhea of turista.

Now that I understand the nature of this problem, I can manage it successfully. By accepting the necessity of a period of intestinal readjustment when I travel, I can minimize the severity and duration of discomfort simply by resting my bowels and avoiding further stresses on them. I fast or eat very lightly, do not take caffeine or other intestinal stimulants and irritants, and avoid drugs like Entero-Vioform, which make everything worse.

Giving Entero-Vioform to travelers is a classic allopathic blunder. That drug is a specific for the protozoal agent of amebic dysentery, an organism not associated with the routine diarrheas of travelers. Moreover, it is an irritating chemical that can cause diarrhea on its own. Long after my travels in 1959, it was recognized to have serious liver and central nervous system toxicity. In fact, it has not been marketed for systemic use for a number of years.

Millions of travelers took this drug on the advice of allopaths (who, in turn, were influenced by the promotional activities of its manufacturer). Not only does Entero-Vioform do nothing to help travelers' diarrhea, it makes the bowel's job of readjustment to new bacteria harder and exposes patients to completely unnecessary risks. Again, the root of this blunder is conceptual.

Fascinated by material agents of disease, allopaths imagine that turista is caused by bad, foreign germs. Their job, then, is to attack those germs, put them out of existence with a potent pharmaceutical weapon. That is simply not the problem or its remedy, and in this case the choice of weapon is even inappropriate, since Entero-Vioform works best for amebas. No doctor ever told me to stop eating when I got turista, nor admitted that foreigners coming to the United States have to deal with the same change in environmental flora and experience the same symptoms.

The fourth example is that of a woman, aged twenty-four, with a long and worrisome history of gynecological problems, including tubal pregnancy, abortion, and recurrent infections. She consulted me a few months after one of the worst of her infections had progressed to peritonitis, requiring hospitalization and massive doses of intravenous antibiotics. She was sent home after four days, and the symptoms disappeared completely a few days after that, but within two days of this apparent recovery, fever recurred, and she was back in the hospital, again with peritonitis. She was once more given antibiotics intravenously — this time, in her words, "enough to kill off all the bacteria on the face of the earth." She finally went home with her digestive system in chaos and with a severe vaginal yeast infection, direct results of the antibiotic treatment.

She called me for help when all the symptoms of pelvic infection returned once more, about four months later. She wanted desperately to avoid another hospitalization. When I talked to her (by telephone — she was many miles away), she had fever, pelvic and abdominal pain, and the same kind of vaginal discharge as during previous episodes. I first made her promise to go to an emergency room if her fever increased after twenty-four hours of trying an alternative approach. She agreed. I then told her to drink at least ten full glasses of water a day, eat very lightly, stay at absolute bed rest, and keep heat on her abdomen. In addition, I required her to meditate on the pain, trying to give it definite form, color, and location with her visual imagination. I urged her to continue this mental exercise for twelve hours with as few interruptions as possible, then report back to me.

In the course of meditating on the pain, she discovered it to be virtually identical to sexual excitement. She also realized it was located in the same part of her body where she experienced both sexual excitement and anxiety and saw that sexual arousal for her had always been bound up with anxiety. These discoveries came as revelations to this patient and started her on an interesting course of self-analysis. She had always had strong sexual impulses, which she had trusted and surrendered to. Now, for the first time, she became aware of her deep ambivalence about sexual arousal. Simultaneously, she understood this ambivalence, with its strong component of anxiety, to be the root of her recurrent gynecological illnesses.

Even in the midst of the present flare-up, these insights made her elated. She now knew the real nature of her problem and the kind of solution it demanded. She would have to sort out her complicated feelings about sex, and although she knew that would be a long process, she also knew that in some way she had begun. Moreover, she was tremendously relieved to know that cure was within her power; she would not have to seek it from doctors, drugs, and hospitals. In fact, her symptoms now decreased quickly, whereas before they had always worsened until she needed outside help. After one week she was back to normal, later got pregnant, and never again had a severe episode of pelvic inflammatory disease.

I recount this case because it made use of a therapeutic technique involving the mind — an imaginary organ to the average allopath. Just what role the meditation and revelatory insights played in this woman's cure I cannot say, but I am sure they contributed to the favorable outcome. By ignoring such methods, allopaths deprive themselves of a host of potentially useful techniques for intervening in disease processes and cannot think what to do when the standard methods fail except to repeat them and repeat them, often at high cost to patients. They would expand their power over health and illness if they made use of nonmaterial factors as well as material ones.

11

Some Medical Heresies:
Osteopathy, Chiropractic, Naturopathy

WHEREVER A SYSTEM OF TREATMENT becomes so established as to merit the name "regular" or "orthodox" medicine, rival systems appear to challenge it. While Hippocrates taught and practiced on Cos, a rival school of medicine grew up on the mainland opposite at Cnidos. The Cnidians insisted on naming diseases, were not that interested in identifying their external causes, and differed from the dominant Hippocratic school in other matters, both practical and theoretical.[1]

In recent times, allopathy has spawned many heretical practices. The strength of unorthodox medicine waxes and wanes depending on the effectiveness of regular doctors in satisfying the needs of patients. During the Age of Heroic Medicine, it was great, fed by intense opposition to the harmful methods then in vogue. In the early part of this century, with widespread public faith in technology and universal admiration for the inventions and discoveries of scientific medicine, it was at an all-time low. Today, medical heresy is again on the increase.

Unorthodox practitioners are now highly visible in most American towns and cities. Many of them advertise, and many attract large and devoted followings of patients. Some M.D.'s, aware of the market that exists for unorthodox therapies, have begun to supplement their allopathic techniques with other methods in order to win back an alienated clientele.

I notice that people who go to unorthodox practitioners usually do not know much about the origins or theories of the systems they use. Such information should figure into the process of making intelligent choices from among the methods of treatment available. This background is relevant to the questions under examination here, particularly as to the nature of treatment and the relationship between treatment and cure. Three medical heresies have survived long enough to become established in their own right. They provide unusual perspectives on allopathic medicine as well as further clues to the answers to my questions.

Osteopathy

Osteopathy ("bone treatment") was the invention of a colorful man named Andrew Taylor Still (1828–1917), who, like Hahnemann before him, was an allopathic doctor disgusted by the methods he had been taught, especially the use of toxic drugs. Also like Hahnemann, Still was deeply religious and convinced that healing was an innate, God-given capacity of the human body. In background and temperament, however, these two successful medical heretics could not have been less alike.

Still was a product of the American frontier, born in a log cabin in Virginia, the son of a Methodist circuit rider and country physician. He grew up in Tennessee and Missouri, served on active duty with the Union Army in the Civil War (he was an ardent Abolitionist), and learned medicine by preceptorship, with only part-time study at a college in Kansas City. Throughout his life, he played the role of crusader and prophet, making passionate friends and equally passionate enemies. To the former he became known affectionately as the Old Doctor.[2]

From his childhood, Still was fascinated by bones. He used to exhume bodies from Indian graves in order to study skeletons. This fascination, combined with an intense desire to find a drugless method of treating disease, led him to the technique of "bony manipulation," which was to form the basis of his new system.

In his autobiography, Still describes a boyhood experience that later prompted his discovery of manipulation therapy:

> One day, when about ten years old, I suffered from a headache. I made a swing of my father's plow-line between two trees; but my head hurt too much to make swinging comfortable, so I let the rope down to about eight or ten inches off the ground, threw

the end of a blanket on it, and I laid down on the ground and used the rope for a swinging pillow. Thus I lay stretched on my back with my neck across the rope. Soon I became easy and went to sleep and got up in a little while with the headache gone. As I knew nothing of anatomy at this time, I took no thought of how a rope could stop a headache and the sick stomach which accompanied it. After the discovery I roped my neck whenever I felt those spells coming on. I followed that treatment for 20 years before the wedge of reason reached my brain and I could see that I had suspended the action of the great occipital nerves, and given harmony to the flow of the arterial blood to and through the veins, and ease was the effect . . .[3]

As a practitioner, Still gave up the use of drugs completely and, instead, tried to promote healing by manipulating bones to allow free circulation of blood and balanced functioning of nerves. The technique he developed was the same used by generations of children to crack their knuckles: placing tension on a joint until an audible click or pop results. Knuckles are relatively easy to crack; some of the larger joints of the body are much harder, but Still found positions and motions to succeed with most of them.

He also found he could get good results in treating sick people by this method alone. Enthusiastic over his discovery, he tried, in 1874, to present his ideas at Baker University in Baldwin, Kansas, but was denied permission to do so. Angered by this rejection, he moved to Kirksville, Missouri, and there opened a medical practice based on osteopathy.

Andrew Taylor Still was not simply curing headaches and stiff necks at this time. Epidemics of serious infectious diseases regularly swept through frontier settlements of the period, and Still took on these problems without hesitation. He used manipulation to treat cases of pneumonia, erysipelas (a bacterial infection of the skin), typhoid fever, and the often-fatal, infectious diarrheas of children, then called flux. He stirred much opposition, both by espousing a heretical method and by never passing up an opportunity to portray regular doctors as poisoners, but he was so successful as a practitioner that he soon attracted a large following.

Here is his own description of his first attempt to treat a case of flux. The year was 1874, and the patient was a four-year-old boy, weak and bleeding from the rectum.

> I placed my hand on the back of the little fellow . . . in the region of the lumbar and found it very warm, even hot, while the abdomen was cold . . . Then the neck and back of his head were very warm, and the face, nose, and forehead cold . . . I began to work at the base of the brain, and thought by pressure and rubbing I could push some of the hot to the cold places. While so doing I found rigid and loose places in the muscles and ligaments of the child's whole spine, while the lumbar region was in a very congested condition. I worked for a few minutes on that philosophy, and then told the mother to report to me the next day, and if I could do anything more for her boy I would cheerfully do so. She came early next morning with the news that her child was well. Flux was prevalent in a large per cent of the families of Macon [Missouri] . . . The lady whose child I had cured brought many people with their sick children to me for treatment. As nearly as I can remember, I had seventeen severe cases of flux in a few days and cured them all without drugs.[4]

Still met each new disease with greater confidence and soon felt he could treat any problem by osteopathic manipulation. He rejected drug treatment as a sacrilege against the body, admitted surgery only as a last resort, and also rejected homeopathy for what he saw as its worthless dispensing of "sugar-coated pills." His practical success brought him patients, money, and fame. In 1892 he began to teach classes in osteopathy at Kirksville, shortly afterward incorporating the American School of Osteopathy, open from the first to blacks and women. From this institution, Still declaimed his doctrine with the style of a fundamentalist preacher and trained men and women as osteopaths.

> What can Osteopathy give us in place of drugs? That is a great question which doctors ask in thunder-tones. Tell them to be seated and listen to a few truths and questions.
> "What will you give in place of drugs?" We have nothing we can give in place of calomel, because Osteopathy does not ruin your teeth, nor destroy the stomach, liver, nor any organ or substance in the system. We cannot give you anything in place of the deadly nightshade, whose poison reaches and ruins the eyes, in sight and shape, and makes tumors great and small. We have

nothing to give in place of aloes, which purge a few times and leave you with unbearable piles for life.

We have nothing to give in place of morphine, chloral, digitalis, veratrine, pulsatilla, and all the deadly sedatives of all schools. We know they will kill and that is all we know about them . . .

In answer to the inquiry, What can you give us in place of drugs? we can give you adjustment of structure but we cannot add or give anything from the material world that would be beneficial to the workings of a perfect machine, that was made and put in running order according to God's judgment, in the construction of all its parts, to add to its form and power day by day, and carry out all exhausted substances that have been made so by wear and motion.

A perfectly adjusted body which will produce pure blood and plenty of it, deliver it on time and in quantity sufficient to supply all demands in the economy of life. This is what the osteopath can give you in the place of drugs if he knows his business.[5]

Like homeopathy, osteopathy became a target of persecution by orthodox medicine as soon as it gained prestige and began to compete successfully for patients. By then homeopathy was relatively respectable and most of its practitioners were eager to make peace with allopaths, whom they joined in denouncing Still's system. Until chiropractic came along to draw some of the fire, osteopathy bore the full brunt of organized allopathy's antiheretical activities.

Once Still was gone and scientific medicine began its triumphal ascendancy in the early twentieth century, osteopaths, like many homeopaths before them, found it in their interest to change their ways in order to gain acceptance with the medical establishment.

I can give no better indication of the extent to which they changed than to point out that Andrew Taylor Still's autobiographical writings first came to my attention in the form of beautifully printed excerpts sent out by a major pharmaceutical company to promote the use of a new, prescription antibiotic. The mailings went to both M.D.'s and D.O.'s (doctors of osteopathy), since both of them now use the same drugs. Poor Dr. Still must be spinning in his grave in the knowledge of what his followers now do in the name of his system. For practical purposes they are indistinguishable from M.D.'s, a fact recognized by the legislatures of several states that have made the two degrees legally equivalent.

There are still osteopathic medical schools and osteopathic hospitals, but, increasingly, allopaths and osteopaths mix freely. The American Osteopathic Association continues to honor Andrew Taylor Still as founder and patriarch of the profession and tries to draw subtle distinctions between D.O.'s and M.D.'s (such as representing osteopaths to be greater believers in the healing power of nature and more attentive to the whole person). The fact is, however, that most osteopaths no longer manipulate, even though they learned the technique in school. They use drugs, surgery, and all the other methods of their allopathic colleagues. The only osteopaths I have met who use manipulation as a primary therapy are rare, elderly ones and an occasional young one, who is suspicious of drugs and "holistically" inclined.

Why did osteopaths give up the method of their prophet? They wanted to jump on the allopathic bandwagon, surely, but they need not have sold out so completely. The answer seems to be that most of them get better results with drugs than they get (or think they could get) with manipulation. Andrew Still had tremendous faith in the method; contemporary osteopaths do not. Moreover, manipulation has received a bad name in orthodox circles from its more recent association with chiropractors and other practitioners now regarded as heretics and quacks.

None of this changes the fact that Still produced cures by manipulation alone, cures of serious diseases. Why the method worked for him and those he first taught but no longer works for today's osteopaths is the key question. Chapter 17 proposes an answer.

Chiropractic

Chiropractic dates from 1895, when its inventor, Daniel David Palmer (1845–1913), discovered what he believed to be the universal cause of all disease and its cure.

Unlike Hahnemann and Still, Palmer was not a doctor, nor was he trained in any profession. He was a grocer, born in Ontario, Canada, who settled in Davenport, Iowa, dabbled in phrenology and spiritualism, then opened what he called a "magnetic healing studio." He felt he had a calling to treat the sick and was obsessed with the search for a single, underlying cause of disease.

One day in September of 1895 he treated in his studio a janitor named Harvey Lillard, who had been deaf for seventeen years. In his autobiography, first published in 1910, Palmer described this event.[6] He noted that the man's deafness had a sudden and curious onset: "When he was exerting himself in a cramped, stooping position, he felt something give way in his back and immediately became deaf."

Palmer examined the man's back and found what he called a "subluxed" (misaligned) vertebra. "I reasoned that if the vertebra was replaced, the man's hearing should be restored. With this object in view a half hour's talk persuaded Mr. Lillard to allow me to replace it."* Palmer had him lie down on his stomach on an examining couch and applied firm pressure to the spine with his hands. "The vertebra moved back into place and soon the man could hear as before." There followed immediately a second success, this time a case of unspecified "heart trouble," also cured by spinal manipulation. On the basis of these two cases, Palmer concluded that "a subluxed vertebra, a vertebral bone, is the cause of 95% of all diseases."[7]

He confided his discovery to a fellow resident of Davenport, the Reverend Samuel Weed, who proposed the name "chiropractic," from Greek roots meaning "done by hand." Before the end of 1895, Palmer had opened the Palmer School of Chiropractic, whose only admission requirement was ability to pay the fee: $450 with a $50 discount for cash.[8]

His most important student was his only son, Bartlett Joshua Palmer (1881–1961), known to all as B.J. In 1906, B.J. and his father were arrested and charged with practicing medicine without a license. The father was tried first and sent to jail; B.J. never came to trial. This incident foreshadowed the very different fortunes of the two men. After Daniel David Palmer got out of jail, he sold his school and business to B.J., then left Iowa and wandered around the United States till his death in 1913. He

*Remember, the man was deaf.

came to hate his son and other chiropractors, died penniless, and left orders that B.J. not be allowed to attend his funeral.

When B.J. died in 1961, he was a multimillionaire who had traveled the world and built chiropractic into a vastly successful empire. He was a commercial genius, the inventor of mail-order diplomas and advertising gimmicks that appalled not only allopaths but also homeopaths and osteopaths. He stated flatly of the Davenport facility: "Our school is on a business, not a professional, basis. We manufacture chiropractors."[9]

B. J. Palmer advertised widely for students, emphasizing the lack of exams or requirements for entrance, encouraged the growth of other schools of questionable reputation, lectured on business psychology, and wrote books with titles like *Radio Salesmanship*. He was fond of making up slogans and having them engraved on the school's walls. One that I like is "Early to bed, early to rise; work like hell and advertise." In a 1952 book called *Questions and Answers About Chiropractic*, he wrote: "Q. What are the principal functions of the spine? A. 1) To support the head; 2) To support the ribs; 3) To support the chiropractor."[10]

Throughout his life, B. J. Palmer affirmed his belief in the pure doctrine of his father: "Chiropractic principle has the vertebral subluxation as the cause of *all* disease; chiropractic practice has the vertebral adjustment as the *cure* of all disease."[11] He, himself, went to M.D.'s when he was sick, however, and some practitioners refused to adhere to the Palmer dogma.

One dissenter was an early convert named Willard Carver, an Oklahoma City lawyer. He set up his own chiropractic school there a few years after the Davenport school opened and developed the idea that chiropractors should use other methods as well as spinal adjustment, including nutritional and physical therapy. His insistence led to a schism in chiropractic between the followers of the Palmer method, who called themselves Straights, and those agreeing with Carver, who became known as Mixers. Each group set up its own school and professional associations, and the division exists to this day, with the Mixers being in the majority, and the Straights still teaching at the original school in Davenport.

B.J.'s facility with high-pressure salesmanship made him an

effective lobbyist for chiropractic. More than any other modern medical heresy, chiropractic has successfully resisted attempts to squelch it and aggressively established itself as a legal, prospering enterprise. By 1925 the profession had great influence in state legislatures, securing licensing in thirty-two of the forty-eight states. (It has since been licensed in all fifty.) It then fought for and won the right to use X-rays and other medical procedures. Chiropractors today cannot perform surgery or prescribe drugs, but they enjoy a great deal of freedom and power and receive reimbursement for their services from both private and governmental insurance agencies. Many patients regard chiropractic as a true alternative to allopathy, on equal footing with it as a scientific system.

Allopaths, of course, are greatly annoyed by that view, since they continue to regard chiropractic as flagrant quackery. One of them has called it "the only legally recognized and licensed superstition in the United States today." The American Medical Association charges that chiropractic education is generally poor, the schools offering little in the way of library or laboratory facilities and few instructors with recognized degrees. It accuses chiropractors of removing patients from scientific treatment and thus endangering their lives, as well as harming them by the direct consequences of manipulation and the overuse of X-rays. Some of these charges are valid, others not.

Chiropractic education has come a long way since the days of B. J. Palmer. On B.J.'s death in 1961, his son, David Daniel Palmer, took over the Davenport school and reorganized it on a more professional basis. He removed B.J.'s books from the library and the slogans from the walls and worked hard to change chiropractic's image, though not its basic philosophy or methods.

The manipulation used by chiropractors is essentially the same as that of osteopaths, but chiropractors restrict it to the spine, while osteopaths — if they manipulate at all — work on all joints, even the relatively immobile joints of the cranium. Manipulation can be scary to someone not used to it, especially sudden motions that crack the vertebrae of the neck, but I do not think it is dangerous. Certainly, it causes nothing near the harm that results from common procedures of orthodox medicine. It also appears to be effective for some patients and some problems, although I have no means of assessing its effectiveness except in an impressionistic way.

Spinal manipulation can immediately relieve the pain of acute musculoskeletal ailments: severe stiff necks, wrenched backs, and so forth, with one session sometimes producing instant and lasting cure. It is probably less successful with chronic problems, such as lower back pain. Allopaths who try to discredit chiropractic argue that manipulation can render patients paraplegic or quadriplegic and can precipitate strokes. I suppose a few instances might be found of paralyses following chiropractic adjustment, but I have never seen evidence of them. Strokes may be a greater risk, especially if the cervical spine is suddenly jerked rather than slowly moved after massage to relax the muscles. Again, I have never seen such mishaps, but I have read of them. They are rare occurrences, much less likely than equivalent accidents from common allopathic procedures performed on the head and neck just for diagnosis.

As for the argument that chiropractors remove sick people from "legitimate" treatment, it is weak. Most patients I know who go to chiropractors for help with serious problems not in the musculoskeletal system do so after exhausting allopathic remedies. The AMA tells tales of children with rare sarcomas (highly malignant cancers of connective tissue) whose parents have placed them in the hands of chiropractors promising cures, only to have the children die rapid and unpleasant deaths. I would like to see documentation of such cases. They are almost certainly very uncommon.

I agree that chiropractors are X-ray happy. They like to impress patients with gigantic films of the whole vertebral column, called "spinographs," that are totally unnecessary. Allopathic radiologists can get all the information they need about the spine with tiny, precise films that require insignificant amounts of radiation compared to a spinograph. Moreover, chiropractors often expose patients to frequent, large doses of X-rays, in order to monitor the changes in the shape of the spine as treatment progresses.

I mentioned in chapter 10 that chiropractors are quite successful in making patients dependent on them. I have never heard of a patient being told he or she has a normal spine on a first visit to one of these practitioners. There are always subluxations. Most patients are told they must come in for regular manipulation to make the adjustments "hold." The tendency of chiropractors to seduce patients into long and costly therapy without promoting self-reliance smacks of the style of B. J. Palmer, who even came up with formulas for determining the number of visits to try for based on a patient's age and annual income.

These failings are incidental to what I see as the central defect of chiropractic. It is not true that all disease results from vertebral misalignment and can be cured by vertebral adjustment. That was the teaching of chiropractic's founder, and it is just plain wrong. Most chiropractors today are Mixers, who employ such other methods as applications of heat and cold, dietary regulation, and prescription of nutritional supplements. Some hold degrees in naturopathy as well; they are D.C.-N.D.'s rather than just D.C.'s. Yet they come from a healing tradition based on a wrong conception, and their Straight colleagues still adhere to the pure dogma of Daniel David Palmer, using spinal manipulation alone to treat all problems.

Manipulation of bones seems to me a good technique to know. I wish I had learned it in medical school. It can be a valuable addition to a doctor's therapeutic repertory, both because it involves a laying-on of hands that can foster productive relationships with patients and because it may improve the circulation of blood and nervous energy to ailing parts of the body. Furthermore, the importance of the spine is probably underrated by allopaths, and even by orthopedists, who are supposed to be the scientific experts on bones. Yoga and other Oriental systems of mind-body development assign highest importance to the spine as the conduit of basic life energy from "out there" to "in here." Many of the practices of physical yoga are intended to improve the function of spinal nerves. Yoga postures practiced over time gradually promote flexibility and good alignment of the vertebral column.

Chiropractors correctly stress the importance of the spine to general health of mind and body, and their manipulative technique may be of real value. It makes no sense, however, to base an entire system of therapy on this technique alone. Chiropractic manipulation should be one method of therapeutic intervention, not an independent and self-sufficient practice.

I must state that I have met some patients who testify to cures of general illnesses as a result of going to chiropractors and more patients who report satisfactory relief of symptoms that regular doctors were unable to treat. Here is one such account from a woman who suffered a disastrous fall:

> When I was thirty years old, in good health, leading an athletic and active life, I fell from a horse that was startled by a sudden noise. I landed on hard ground and hit hard, almost entirely on my lower back. My neck snapped back at the same time, rendering me semiconscious for nearly half an hour.
>
> The consequences of the injury were devastating. I suffered impairment of vision and hearing, recurrent dizziness, some memory loss, and persistent disabling pain in my head, jaw, neck, and shoulder, along with back pain that radiated into my arms and legs.
>
> I sought help from M.D.'s immediately after the accident — first from an internist, who found no broken bones or "permanent damage," just "soft-tissue trauma." He sent me to eye and ear specialists and a neurosurgeon, who concurred in the diagnosis and felt that my nerve and muscle impairments would resolve. The treatments they prescribed were a cervical collar, a drug for pain (containing a barbiturate), and physical therapy.
>
> I was sent to a dentist for the jaw pain. He sent me to a periodontist, who made me wear a device to correct my bite. I was sent to an orthopedic surgeon for my hip pain. He recommended physical therapy directed at the lower back.
>
> For fourteen months I remained in constant, severe pain, especially in my neck. During the next four months, as the treatment continued, the pain began to spread along the entire length of my back. Eighteen months after the injury, in great frustration, I ended my relationships with all the medical doctors I had been seeing and went to a highly recommended chiropractor.
>
> After examining me and taking X-rays, this man began to treat me with a series of physical manipulations of my back, pelvis, and head. During one early session, he told me he had to perform a major adjustment of my neck. He turned my neck to the side in such a way that it made a loud popping noise. This movement hurt severely, but almost immediately afterward I was aware that

the pain I had been living with since the accident was gone and that I could move my neck somewhat freely, also for the first time since the accident. During that day, I was distinctly aware of a significant improvement in my memory and in my general feeling of comfort and wellness.

Over the next two months, the chiropractor continued to manipulate my back and neck, which resulted in progressive improvement in all aspects of my health. He then told me he would begin to use "craniology" to correct displacements in the bones of my skull. This treatment decreased the sensations of pressure and pain in my head and improved my mental function greatly (from the level it had fallen to after the injury). It was definitely hard on me, too, in that I lost weight and had to rest frequently during the two months these cranial sessions went on.

Overall, however, I would say that while I was under the care of medical doctors I regressed continuously and did not ever improve. As soon as I changed to chiropractic care, I began to improve right away and soon after improved dramatically. The experience has been fascinating and also very frustrating, as you might guess. For the first ten months after being injured, while in treatment with a variety of M.D.'s, I spent about twenty-two hours of each day in bed, unable even to read because my mind was working so poorly. Chiropractic has not been a sure thing — sometimes the treatments caused improvements and sometimes they did not — but had I not discovered it as an option, I think I would have continued to deteriorate to the point of total disability.

I wish I had hard data on the frequency of chiropractic successes, but I know of no good studies by disinterested investigators. Why chiropractic succeeds at all in treating medical problems other than stiff necks and backs is a crucial question. The fact that a therapeutic system based on a wrong idea can sometimes produce real cures must be taken into account by any comprehensive theory of health and medicine.

Naturopathy

Naturopathic doctors (N.D.'s) sometimes say their practice can trace its lineage back to Hippocrates and the esoteric science of ancient Egypt, but it seems to derive more immediately from the European tradition of health spas that flowered in the eighteenth and nineteenth centuries. As a formal system of treatment, it dates back only to 1900, when its founder, Benedict Lust (1872–1945) established the first naturopathic college. Naturopathy is not only the newest of the major medical heresies, it is also the least organized, both in theory and practice. Lacking a strong political arm, it has never developed the professional structure of osteopathy and chiropractic and is licensed in fewer than one quarter of the states of the United States.

I have found it difficult to locate information on the history of naturopathy or Dr. Lust, and I find the definitions of the system by its proponents to be unhelpfully vague. For example, a naturopathic college in California tells us that

> the science of naturopathic medicine is an ever-expanding body of knowledge drawn from diverse traditional and modern sources. It is a record of observation and research from many cultures throughout history. Included in this science are the disciplines common to all healing arts — a thorough study of the human organism, how it is influenced by all aspects of its environment, and techniques of discovering the nature of disease processes. Naturopathic physicians apply the latest research in all branches of medical science and technology to their field — from discoveries of new facts about human physiology, biochemistry, and nutrition to the most modern diagnostic tools and techniques.

The ratio of hard information to number of words in that passage is quite low; it is typical of statements about naturopathy. I think the vagueness reflects a lack of theoretical coherence to the system, related also to a lack of professional coherence or power.

Benedict Lust was an M.D. from Germany who emigrated to the United States in 1892. Like other medical heretics, he was dissatisfied with orthodox practice. Convinced of the innate healing powers of nature, he looked for more natural, less harmful methods of treatment than surgery and strong drugs.

German-speaking Europe is the ancestral homeland of naturopathy, for Lust took his inspiration from individuals and traditions in that part of the world. Germany, Austria, and Switzerland have long been famous for their health resorts and curative spas. These centers were still very active when Lust was looking for alternative therapies, and they caught his attention. Prominent at them were various water cures that took such diverse forms as soaks in natural hot springs, applications of hot and cold water to parts of the body, and mineral-water fasts. Toward the end of the last century, a number of practitioners advanced water cures as new scientific treatment, giving them the modern-sounding name hydrotherapy.

One advocate of the healing power of water was Father Sebastian Kneipp (1821–1897), an Austrian priest who cured himself of a supposedly fatal lung condition by plunging into ice-cold water every day for many months. He got the idea from the writings of a countryman, Vincenz Priessnitz (1799–1851), a farmer who believed that bacteria disliked cold more than heat, because cold generally inhibited animal breeding. Kneipp recovered fully and began to teach a natural, curative system based on ice-cold baths and barefoot walks in grass and cold streams. Later, he also advocated the use of light, fresh air, and herbs.[12]

Benedict Lust adopted the Kneipp water cure as a principal method of treating illness. When he came to America in 1892, his purpose was to practice and teach this form of hydrotherapy. The Kneipp method attracted an assortment of medical heretics: homeopaths, herbalists, and lay practitioners who believed in natural healing. Allopaths did not account for a high proportion of this ill-defined group. Unlike homeopathy and osteopathy, naturopathic medicine never seriously challenged allopathy by drawing converts from the orthodox ranks. Yet its main proponent, Lust, was a physician, and the system has never been as distant from regular medicine as chiropractic has.

In 1900 a committee of Kneipp practitioners decided to broaden their practice to include all the natural methods espoused by the assorted supporters of hydrotherapy: botanical remedies, homeopathy, nutritional therapy, psychology, massage, and the new systems of bony manipulation. A German homeopath, Dr. John H. Scheel, proposed the name naturopathy to describe the practice of this coalition. Shortly afterward, Benedict Lust opened the American School of Naturopathy in New York City, graduating the first class in 1902.

Naturopathy did not spring from a unified doctrine, nor was

it launched by a charismatic prophet like Hahnemann, Still, or Palmer. It emerged slowly and without clear definition from an informal grouping of people who shared certain beliefs about health and medicine. There are naturopaths today who mainly manipulate bones, others who massage muscles, others who prescribe pills, others who use herbs, others who still favor hydrotherapy and applications of heat and cold, others who encourage fasting and colonic irrigation, others who use acupuncture, others who use forms of homeopathy, others who use several of these methods in combination.

All naturopaths reject surgery and the strong drugs of the allopath except as last resorts. Speaking in 1925, Benedict Lust said, "Most people die from the effects of wrong living and drugs . . . Most diseases and chronic sicknesses are only aggravated by the use of medicine."[13] Naturopaths also believe in the vital natural force, the healing power of nature, the *medicatrix vis naturae* of Hippocrates. They try to stimulate healing from within and favor gentle methods of stimulation over harsh ones. They do not agree, however, on which methods are best and appear to have no clear, shared theories on the nature of illness.

In some ways, the original naturopaths were glorified hygienists, who felt that clean living was the way to good health — hence the emphasis on fresh air, good diet, water, light, herbs, and other simple measures. Our word *hygiene* comes from Hygeia, the Greek goddess of health, daughter of Asklepios. Regular physicians invoke her when they take the Hippocratic oath, which opens with the magnificent line, "I swear by Apollo the Healer and by Asklepios, by Hygeia and Panacea,* and by all the gods and goddesses, making them my witnesses, that I will fulfill according to my power and judgment this oath and covenant."

Hygeia and Asklepios represent two poles of thinking about health and medicine, a point made clearly by medical writer and philosopher René Dubos:

> For the worshippers of Hygeia, health is the natural order of things, a positive attribute to which men are entitled if they govern

---

*Asklepios's other daughter presides over the materia medica; her name means "all-heal."

their lives wisely. According to them, the most important function of medicine is to discover and teach the natural laws which will ensure a man a healthy mind in a healthy body. More skeptical, or wiser in the ways of the world, the followers of Asklepios believe that the chief role of the physician is to treat disease, to restore health by correcting any imperfections caused by accidents of birth or life.[14]

As a collection of nonharmful methods oriented toward the Hygeian pole, naturopathy can offer a refreshing balance to the aggressive, invasive, and unnatural practices of modern allopathy. Regrettably, many naturopaths have begun to worship Asklepios in their own way, falling under the spell of science and technology.

It was naturopathy's misfortune to come on the scene late — just as technological medicine began its meteoric rise. Naturopathy never got the support of a public outraged by the heroic practices of the early and middle 1800s and has always been overshadowed by osteopathy and chiropractic. In fact, until recently, most N.D.'s have also been chiropractors. The education and training of these chiropractor-naturopaths leave much to be desired.

In the past few years, naturopathic schools have become better, graduating a new generation of pure N.D.'s whose preclinical education is much more thorough than that of chiropractors. At the same time, however, some of these younger naturopaths, in an effort to appear more scientific, tend to embrace gimmicks, gadgets, and the trappings of medical technology, a significant departure from the founders of the system and from Hygeian principles.

Many naturopaths now use a diagnostic procedure called hair-shaft analysis, for example. They send off a sample of a patient's hair to a laboratory for analysis, getting the results back as impressive computer print-outs that give figures for many nutrients and minerals and indicate departures from normal values. The practitioner then recommends dietary changes or nutrient and mineral supplements on the basis of the test.

In principle, hair-shaft analysis is appealing, because it is non-invasive and might be able to provide information about nutritional and biochemical abnormalities in other tissues. In practice, it is suspect. First of all, evidence for correlations between hair chemistry and that of the rest of the body is lacking. Even if the test results are meaningful, I do not think anyone can make valid interpretations of them. A high level of copper in hair does not necessarily indicate an excess of copper in the living tissues of the body and may have no significance to health and the management of illness. Furthermore, I am not convinced that hair-shaft analysis is accurate. One of the few studies of it found that different laboratories reported different results from the same hair sample and that in some instances different results came back from the same laboratory for separate specimens of the same hair, labeled as if they came from more than one patient.[15]

Given the uncertainties of this diagnostic technique, it is disappointing to see naturopaths rely on it so much. Some of them base all of their treatment on the results, putting patients on bizarre dietary regimens that may have nothing to do with biochemical reality or the problems that made the patients seek help in the first place. Naturopaths who act in this way are no different from allopaths who rely heavily on laboratory results. Both are treating abnormalities on paper rather than improving health. The appeal of hair-shaft analysis and other unorthodox procedures clothed in the forms of scientific medicine is obvious. They fascinate patients and make naturopaths feel more like "real" doctors.

Why today's naturopaths find it necessary to cast about for more powerful methods of diagnosis and treatment is an interesting question. It points up the dilemma of the natural healer in a world where faith in science is stronger than faith in nature. I know one young naturopath who has just enrolled in conventional medical school to work for an M.D. For several years he practiced with his N.D., relying on massage, bony manipulation, herbal treatment, and a form of homeopathy. He says he is sure he will always use manipulation because he has seen it produce good results. As a believer in the healing power of nature, he wants to encourage it by effective and nonharmful means. He abandoned naturopathic practice for two reasons. The weakness of naturopathy as an organized profession left him feeling isolated, and his results in general were not good enough. He wants to learn more powerful methods.

There is an abundance of testimonials on record about dramatic reversals of illness by nature cures of one sort or another. Father Kneipp's story is a classic example. I had one patient, a twenty-five-year-old man, who gave me another. He was traveling in southern Mexico, was exposed to infectious hepatitis along with several companions, all of whom later developed typical symptoms of the disease and had the usual long course of recovery. There is no orthodox treatment for hepatitis other than bed rest, good diet, and avoidance of additional stress to the inflamed liver; hepatitis can make people ill for weeks or months. In young children, however, the disease may be as mild as a light cold, and some adults become much sicker with it than others.

The first symptoms of hepatitis are nonspecific and common to many viral infections: malaise, loss of appetite, weakness. There follow specific symptoms: liver pain, intolerance to certain foods and drugs (notably cigarettes), and manifestations of liver obstruction, such as dark brown urine, clay-colored stools, and jaundice that is first apparent in the whites of the eyes. My patient reported that his companions took no action when they started to feel ill. They did not rest, continued to eat heavily, and soon were on their backs, unable to get out of bed, strongly jaundiced, and in great discomfort. They remained sick for many weeks.

The young man came down with the early symptoms after his friends and realized at once what was happening. He stopped eating, went to a hot spring with a large supply of bottled mineral water, and did nothing but rest, fast, soak for long periods in the hot spring, and force a great deal of bottled water through his system. He had one episode of dark urine and light stools, but the normal colors quickly returned, and he never became jaundiced. After forty-eight hours of this regimen, he began eating fruit and cautiously resumed activity. He had no further symptoms and attributes his cure to early intervention by natural methods that strengthened his body's defenses.

Nature cures have this potential to reverse illness, even very serious illness. They illustrate the principle that the body has innate healing abilities, and they should receive more attention from all medical practitioners, especially allopaths.

As the basis of a system of practice, however, nature cures do not seem to stand up well in the modern world. Naturopathy is not a strong competitor in the rivalry of available therapies, and to attract and hold patients today, naturopaths have to use gimmicks and gadgets. The healing power of nature is real. Why is it unable to sustain a formal system of medical practice as the twentieth century comes to a close?

12

Chinese Medicine

I FIND IT AMUSING to see Oriental medicine sometimes included in lists of "nontraditional therapies." Unorthodox it may be by Western standards, but I cannot think of a more traditional therapeutic system. Chinese medicine began at least three thousand years ago, developed into a true science that flowered between the tenth and thirteenth centuries, and, even after hundreds of years of decline, is not only important in China today but even resurgent.

Of course, many indigenous forms of medicine exist in contemporary Asia, from the ayurvedic practice of India* to shamanism and a variety of local healing cults, but traditional Chinese practice has dominated the East, extending to Tibet, Japan, central Asia, and now even to the West, in keeping with renewed interest in alternatives to allopathy.

No medical system is less like allopathy than the Chinese. It is rooted in ideas and conceptions totally different from those of Western science and, really, is quite irreconcilable with it, despite ongoing attempts at reconciliation, such as the search for unique electrophysical characteristics of acupuncture points. Yet Chinese medicine seems to complement its Western counterpart in an elegant way and certainly has much to teach us about the nature of healing and treatment and the subtle relationship between them.

Being logical thinkers, Chinese theoreticians have constructed a precisely articulated body of medical theory beginning with

*A system based on Ayur-Veda, one of the sacred texts of the ancient Aryans. It stresses dietary regimens and treatment with botanical drugs.

philosophical concepts they take as axioms. The particular philosophy that forms the basis of the system is Taoism. For Taoists, health is a manifestation of the harmony of heaven, attained by proper balance of internal and external forces. Taoists find unity in the diversity of natural phenomena by postulating a basic, universal energy underlying all of them. The Chinese call this energy *ch'i* and believe that it flows into and through the human body and all its parts. Health requires that each organ have just the right amount of *ch'i* to perform its function. An excess or deficiency of *ch'i* will result in malfunction of an organ and imbalance of the whole body, which is disease.

In essence, diagnosis in Chinese medicine is concerned with identifying the location and nature of energy imbalances: which organs they affect and whether they are excesses or deficiencies. Treatment is then a matter of correcting the problems by bringing more *ch'i* to deficient organs and drawing it away from ones with too much.

Taoists proceed from a consideration of unity to a fascination with polarity: from the concept of "1" to the concept of "2." They identify two opposite and complementary qualities to all aspects of being and call them *yang* and *yin*. Yang is positive, expansive, masculine, light, big, having the nature of heaven, of day, of the left side and surface of an object, of wood and fire, and so forth. Yin is negative, contractive, feminine, dark, small, having the nature of earth, of night, of the right side and interior of an object, of metal and water. All substances, objects, times, places, and other aspects of creation are mixtures of these qualities. Proper classification of them enables a practical Taoist to combine them in ways that promote general balance. For example, an overly yang person should eat more yin food.

Chinese medical doctors classify the organs of the body as yang and yin, hollow ones being yang and solid ones yin. All foods and medicinal herbs are so classified, along with all other variables relevant to health and treatment.

In addition, Chinese medical philosophers emphasize a five-stage process of dynamic evolution in phenomenal reality, often called the five-element theory and symbolized by wood, fire, earth, metal, and water. All substances and objects are referable to these five elements, alone or in combination, and, again, the

Chinese rigorously classify foods, drugs, and organs of the body according to this scheme. Thus the spleen and stomach are assigned to the realm of "earth," while the lung and large intestine belong to "metal."

We usually think of elements as unchanging, but for the Chinese these five categories are in a constant process of evolution, whereby one element controls another while giving rise to a third according to a fixed and cyclic pattern. Wood controls earth (as trees stand upon the ground) and is controlled in turn by metal (which can fell the biggest trees); wood also generates fire (when it burns) and is in turn generated by water (which makes trees grow). Since each bodily organ is assigned to one of these elements, this scheme pictures the functional relationships among the organs. The liver (wood) controls the spleen (earth) and is controlled by the lung (metal); it also generates the activity of the heart (fire), and its own activity is generated by the kidney (water). These relationships indicate the direction of flow of *ch'i* energy from one organ to another (see the diagram on page 146).

The Chinese identify twelve organs, but here the divergence from Western conceptions is extreme — a fact obscured by inaccurate translation. The Chinese term *tsang*, usually rendered as "organ," means something like "sphere of function" and does not necessarily equate with any object known to an anatomist. When Chinese doctors diagnose an excess of *ch'i* in the liver, they may not be talking about the liver as we know it but about a sphere of bodily function that may include all or part of the anatomical liver and whose activities may or may not correlate with Western scientific ideas of liver function. In fact, two of the twelve Chinese organs have no anatomical correspondence at all; they are called "triple heater" and "circulation-sex," to the bafflement of those who would like to find neat equivalencies between East and West.[1]

Chinese custom prohibits autopsies. Cutting into a dead body was unthinkable in ancient China and still is for many of its people today. Consequently, traditional Chinese doctors had to proceed without detailed knowledge of internal anatomy and never embraced surgery as a therapeutic method. They concentrated on function rather than form; hence their identification

The Chinese Conception of Energy Circulation
Through the Body

MAXIMUM ENERGY (CH'I)

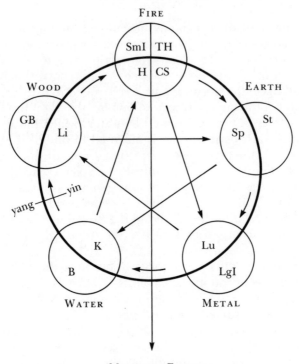

MINIMUM ENERGY

	= control cycle		= generational cycle

SmI	= Small Intestine	H	=	Heart
TH	= Triple Heater	CS	=	Circulation-Sex
St	= Stomach	Sp	=	Spleen
LgI	= Large Intestine	Lu	=	Lung
B	= Bladder	K	=	Kidney
GB	= Gall Bladder	Li	=	Liver

of twelve spheres of function that correspond imperfectly to anatomical organs with the same names. Unequipped to assess pathological changes in the internal structure of the body, they learned instead to recognize and correct disturbances of body functions.

The theory of Chinese medicine is concerned mainly with the energy mechanics of the body: the pathways and directions of flow of energy from "organ" to "organ" and ways to influence it. These pathways are deduced from the theory of yang-yin polarity and that of the five elements (or five evolving phases). There is one more important theoretical concept in the system: namely, that the flows of energy in the interior of the body are mirrored in flows on the surface. This is a crucial point, because the deep flows are inaccessible to direct medical intervention, but the superficial flows can be changed — by acupuncture — and doing so will indirectly affect the energetics of ailing organs. Chinese doctors also believe that energy imbalances in internal organs are reflected in changes of superficial pulses that can be felt by a trained observer and used as a basis for diagnosis.

The traditional Chinese doctor makes a diagnosis by questioning, observing, and listening to the patient, and by feeling the pulses. Answers to questions about symptoms and findings of abnormalities in breath sounds, skin color and texture, or general bodily appearance and odor may provide clues to the location of problems in one or more of the twelve organs and may indicate its nature in terms of imbalances in yang-yin or in the five elements. Confirmation of these clues and indications must be sought with pulse diagnosis.

Chinese pulse reading is to allopathic pulse reading as the *Mona Lisa* is to a newspaper cartoon. As an allopath, I am trained to palpate (feel) the pulse of the radial artery at the wrist, primarily to count it and note whether it is regular or irregular. It does not matter which wrist I use, and though I may write down a word or two about the strength or quality of the pulse, my interest is limited to rate and rhythm. It is not very hard to learn to read a pulse in this fashion; anyone can do it with a little practice.

The Chinese doctor also uses the radial artery pulse at the wrist, but he feels it with the first three fingers of his hand, on both wrists, and with both light and firm pressure. He learns to distinguish a pulse under each finger at each level of pressure and so records twelve separate pulses, six on each wrist. He believes each correlates with the activity of a specific sphere of bodily function — "spleen," "large intestine," "circulation-sex," and so on.

Chinese pulse diagnosis is a highly refined art, difficult to master, requiring years of attentive practice and careful correlation with symptoms. One must learn to distinguish subtle qualities of each pulse, not just its rate and rhythm, and also to assess how each fits in with the whole. One practitioner I met told me he thinks of the pulses as a twelve-piece orchestra and tries to determine which instruments are playing out of tune.

By means of questions, observation, and the refined and subtle art of pulse diagnosis — all noninvasive techniques — the Chinese doctor determines which organs are malfunctioning and whether the problems are excesses or deficiencies of energy.

Methods to correct the problems commonly include massage, herbal drugs, and dietary regimens, with selection of foods and herbs based on yang-yin and five-element theory. A patient who appears deficient in metal may be given a metal herb; if the problem is in a particular metal organ, like the lung, selection of the drug will be restricted to those metal herbs believed to have special affinities with the lung.

In addition to these measures, the Chinese doctor relies on a powerful and unique therapeutic method — acupuncture. It is the insertion of needles into special points on the body in order to draw energy to or from internal organs by changing the related flows on the surface. Acupuncture is an ancient technique, its origins lost in antiquity. Before the end of the Stone Age in what is now China, people may have used stone needles to treat illness and had identified specific points through which symptoms could be influenced. Much later, these points were referred to the twelve organs and connected in lines, usually called meridians.

Each organ has a superficial meridian with many numbered points. The meridians end and begin at the fingers and toes, where the polarity of *ch'i* is said to change. Most needling is done below the elbows and knees, because energy circulation is most easily influenced near the origins and terminations of the meridians.

The acupuncture points may be stimulated both by needles and by heat. In the latter case, a bit of dried plant material is burned on the point, a procedure known as moxibustion (after *moxa*, the name of the material). Identification of the points is based on strict anatomical criteria and requires precision and practice. Even very slight errors in needle placement will result in ineffective treatment. Needles are usually inserted quickly in one or more points and left in place for several minutes. Sometimes the acupuncturist will move or twirl them to increase the stimulation.

Selection of points to needle is dictated by the pattern of energy flows outlined above. If the liver is diagnosed to have excess *ch'i*, energy may be drawn away from it by stimulating the heart sphere (using the generational cycle by which wood gives rise to fire) or by stimulating the spleen sphere (using the control cycle, where wood controls earth). If heart stimulation is decided upon, the acupuncturist selects a point or points on the heart meridian believed to connect with the liver; needling them will draw energy from the liver meridian to the heart meridian, and this change in superficial flow of *ch'i* will then be reflected sympathetically in the more important internal flow. The end result should be improved function of the liver as it regains balance.

Chinese doctors follow many rules in using acupuncture, based on their understanding of it as a means of manipulating a real form of energy. They will not perform it if outside temperature exceeds body temperature or during the time of the full moon or during lightning storms, for example, because they say these conditions disturb the process. Such rules do not make the method any more comprehensible to Western scientists.

Allopathic doctors have known about acupuncture for a long time, but until very recently regarded it as little different from sticking pins in wax dolls for purposes of black magic. When I was in medical school in the mid-1960s acupuncture was a laughable topic if it came up at all, proof of how far rational science had brought us from a former age of superstition.

How this attitude changed is an interesting story. If one event was responsible, it was front-page publicity in 1972 about the success of acupuncture in relieving postoperative pain. A well-known *New York Times* reporter underwent an emergency appendectomy during the first official visit by Americans to China after the Communist revolution. He told the Western world that Chinese needles really worked. That publicity created an enormous demand for acupuncture in the United States, probably much of it from patients who were fed up with orthodox treatment and hungry for an alternative. Not until American doctors realized that large numbers of patients were more willing to pay money for acupuncture than for regular remedies did they take the Chinese method seriously and begin to investigate it.

Ironically, it is a nontraditional aspect of acupuncture that has chiefly caught the fancy of the West: its use for control or elimination of pain. Acupuncture anesthesia is interesting but not central to Chinese medicine, where the main purpose of inserting needles is to effect changes in body energetics.

A great many acupuncturists in the United States stick needles into people today, but little of this activity is consistent with traditional Chinese practice. Laws vary from state to state as to who may do it and what training they require. Few acupuncturists here are trained in Chinese ways. Fewer are able to practice pulse diagnosis. Most use the needles for pain control. Many are unskilled in correct identification of the points, and some use bizarre placements of needles and such gimmicks as electrical stimulation through them. I met one elderly obstetrician in Oregon who packed his waiting room by offering acupuncture to old patients with rheumatism and arthritis. While I watched him at work, connecting the needles to an array of wires and lights, he told me he did not think it was all that important where he put them. "Sometimes I just stick them right into the joint," he said, "and it doesn't seem to make any difference."

Acupuncture anesthesia certainly works for many people. I know a number of dentists who find they can deaden pain sufficiently to drill teeth just by needling a point on the hand. They no longer use nitrous oxide gas or injections of local anesthetics in most of their patients. Moreover, the scientific credibility of the procedure has increased enormously with the recent discovery that the effect can be neutralized by prior treatment with narcotic antagonists — drugs that block the actions of opiates.

This finding suggests that acupuncture anesthesia is mediated by the brain's own narcotics — the endorphins — a group of chemicals I will discuss in connection with placebo responses.

It seems to me that scientific medicine cannot easily go beyond this peripheral application of acupuncture because the more important, traditional uses derive from non-Western concepts. The essential problem is Chinese emphasis on "energy," a non-material quantity that looks hopelessly vague and mystical to the average allopath. I find it hard to talk about *ch'i* or yang and yin with medical doctors. They often ask, "Just what do you mean by 'energy'?" Of course, energy has a precise meaning in physics: it is the ability to do work, and it should not be difficult to see body processes as energetic phenomena — the beating of the heart, movement of intestines, manufacture of hormones and enzymes, and so forth. Nevertheless, most proponents of scientific medicine cannot understand this simple concept. Their rigid materialism and habit of thinking of medicine as separate from the deep concerns of philosophy and religion make the Chinese system of therapeutics inaccessible, seemingly unscientific and irrelevant.

In fact, Chinese medicine has much to teach allopaths and scientists.

Assessment of the effectiveness of this system is complicated by its present degenerate nature. After its golden age ended in the thirteenth century, as a result of general changes in Chinese society, traditional medicine went into a long decline, bottoming out a hundred years ago. It became grossly contaminated by superstitious and magical practices and divorced from the pure and powerful philosophy that spawned it. Most of its modern practitioners do not understand its theories and so cannot use them as a basis for intuitive and artful therapy; instead, they practice a sort of cookbook medicine, uninspired and unguided by sound ideas.

Only very recently has the Chinese government encouraged traditional medicine and elevated it to a status that can attract good minds. For much of this century, Chinese obsession with modernization produced a contempt for the system and a strong desire to replace it with Western scientific methods. Traditional Chinese medicine may be quite effective with certain health problems, but it cannot be judged in its present form. Still, we should consider that it has survived an impressive test of time, enduring over millennia as the principal system of health care for a large population admired for its achievements in art, social organization, technological innovation, and many other areas of human endeavor.

The aims of Chinese medicine are lofty, distinct from those of allopathy, and worth understanding. Because it is chiefly concerned with function and the energy economy of the body, it is better equipped to deal with illness in its earliest stages — indeed, in stages so early that Western doctors might not be able to detect them. Chinese doctors make a clear distinction between "invisible" and "visible" illness. They say all visible illness is preceded by invisible illness. The idea is that imbalances of energy in the body, if allowed to persist, will eventually cause changes in the material structure of the body — changes that are more serious and much harder to reverse. By correcting excesses and deficiencies of energy in vital spheres of function, the acupuncturist prevents invisible illness from becoming visible; that is his primary responsibility.

In chapter 6, I explained what seems to me to be a self-evident principle of health and illness under the heading "Subtle Manifestations of Illness Precede Gross Ones." The more observant and intuitive allopathic doctors are in their diagnoses, the better they will be at detecting disease in its early, subtle stages, when treatment is surer and drastic intervention less necessary. Even the most materialistic allopaths regularly see cases of disease so subtle that no material changes are detectable. Physical examination, X-rays, and lab tests are all normal, but the patient knows something is wrong. There may be pain, disturbance of sleep, mood change, abnormal digestion, or other symptoms. Western doctors even label many of these cases "functional," correctly suggesting that they have no measurable structural correlates, but incorrectly implying that they are unimportant or "all in the mind." Actually, they are likely to be in the immaterial body rather than the material one, or, as the Chinese would say, in the pattern of energy circulation and use. This area is precisely the focus of Chinese diagnosis and treatment.

Emphasis on detection and treatment of the subtle stages of

illness gives traditional Chinese doctors more power than their Western counterparts to practice real preventive medicine. Allopaths talk about prevention but occupy themselves with management of acute crises. The Chinese view is well expressed in a book dating at least from the early Han period (206 B.C. to A.D. 25), the *Huang Ti Nei Ching Su Wen*, translated into English under the curious title *The Yellow Emperor's Classic of Internal Medicine*. It is the oldest medical book extant, and parts of it may come from truly ancient times.

The passage I refer to is:

> Hence the sages did not treat those who were already ill; they instructed those who were not yet ill. They did not want to rule those who were already rebellious; they guided those who were not yet rebellious. This is the meaning of the entire preceding discussion [about the importance of harmonizing human life with the changing seasons]. To administer medicines to diseases which have already developed and to suppress revolts which have already developed is comparable to the behavior of those persons who begin to dig a well after they have become thirsty, and of those who begin to cast weapons after they have already engaged in battle. Would these actions not be too late?[2]

This is an eminently sane medical application of Lao-tzu's memorable line: "The biggest problem in the world could have been solved when it was small." The traditional Chinese doctor might offer this paraphrase: the most advanced organic illness in the world could have been cured when it was still functional.

Potentially, Chinese medicine complements ours. The Chinese system should be more successful with functional illnesses and those whose lack of associated structural change puts them out of reach of allopathic methods of diagnosis and treatment. Allopathy, in turn, is more successful with advanced illness, where material changes are marked and responsive only to more drastic techniques of intervention. Possibly, an ideal interaction of the two systems is closer to reality in China today than in any other time and place. The present government of the People's Republic encourages the simultaneous practice of the two, and in some hospitals patients can choose the kind of treatment they want, with the advice of doctors trained in both schools.[3]

Chinese medicine also has much to teach us about the reality of subtle factors in health and illness. Emphasis on a universal energy is an example. Identification of points on the body surface that permit modification of symptoms is another. Some Western scientists have shown acupuncture points to be highly localized areas of low electrical resistance, but the whole scheme of points and meridians just will not fit neatly into the Western conceptual framework, and its relationship to anatomy and physiology looks completely opaque. Yet Chinese doctors make practical use of it, as they do of subtle qualities of pulses not recognized as real by allopaths.

I find here a suggestion that more may be real than meets Western eyes. Just because we cannot detect, perceive, or measure forces and factors Chinese doctors say are important in managing illness does not automatically mean they do not exist. In view of the successes of Chinese medicine, we should keep open minds and continue to try to detect, perceive, and measure. Furthermore, if scientific doctors are able to learn to perceive the reality of these subtle factors, they should then be willing to consider the possibility that others exist, too — like the healing power of nature, or human energy fields that influence the growth of plants, or the "electric" and "magnetic" currents that yogis say flow along the spinal cord, or the human aura that some persons claim to see. Some of these ideas may turn out to be sheer nonsense, but we will never know till we approach them without prejudice and try to share the experiences of those who experience them.

One account I have collected of a successful use of Chinese medicine comes from an allopath, chief of clinical pharmacology in a San Francisco hospital at the time of the event. He had been studying acupuncture as a possible aid in managing heroin withdrawal. Since his problem was organic, not simply functional, his story is all the more interesting.

> While we were preparing our study, several of my associates urged me to try acupuncture for treatment of my right knee, which had been swollen for at least six weeks. I was in excellent general health, and X-rays of my knee were normal, but the pain had prevented me from running my customary five to seven miles a day. All of my attempts to correct the problem had failed, so I

agreed to try. Disposable acupuncture needles were inserted into my right and left ears at the "knee points." The procedure was painless; when the needles were twirled, there was a slight stinging sensation. Several sticks were made in the "knee region" of each ear. The needles remained in place for about fifteen minutes.

I sensed no immediate change and was anxious to go out and prove the procedure ineffective. To my surprise I ran a brisk seven miles. I had been totally unable to run for six weeks. I noted that although the knee was stiff and the rest of my body was sore afterward, I was able to move the knee with much less discomfort than before. After this one treatment, the chronic knee effusion [swelling due to fluid accumulation in the joint] disappeared in two days, and I was able to resume my regular running.

This experience brought home to me how little we know of healing, whether produced by orthodox or unorthodox practices.

13

Shamanism, Mind Cures, and Faith Healing

THE THERAPIES about to be described operate on the mental sphere, either directly by requiring some sort of profession of belief in healing, or indirectly by convincing patients that powerful forces for improvement have been set in motion. They all spring from the common ground of medicine and religion.

Shamanism

Shamanism is the traditional religion of primitive hunting-and-gathering peoples throughout the world. In its purest form, it is native to central and northern Asia, whence it came to the New World in the migrations that populated North and South America. Shamans abound in the Indian tribes of the Americas and still are found in Siberia as well. In Australia, Africa, and the rest of Asia, similar practitioners exist. Whether you call them true shamans, or medicine men, or witch doctors, or voodoo priests, they have much in common with their American counterparts. All act as doctors for their own people as well as for outsiders who travel to consult them.

Shamanism revolves around highly trained individuals who mediate personally between the ordinary world and other worlds of spirits and supernatural forces. Shamans leave their bodies and visit realms not accessible to most people in order to diagnose and solve problems. They make use of altered states of consciousness for these journeys, calling upon helper spirits, especially of animals, to protect themselves from harm and extend their perceptions. In Siberia and the Americas, hallucinogenic plants are favored tools for changing consciousness, with drumming, chanting, and dancing used to direct the travels. In the rest of the world, drumming, chanting, and dancing are mostly used without the aid of drugs.

Shamans learn their techniques by apprenticeship to other shamans, often paying high fees for the instruction and making major commitments of time. Some begin their training as children or adolescents. Most are men, because women in primitive societies are usually too occupied with the tasks of child rearing and crop tending to devote the necessary time to shamanistic study and practice. Women shamans are not unknown, however. In some cultures they are powerful and distinguished.

The rest of a tribe usually regards the shaman with a mixture of awe, fear, and respect. Their lives and the survival of the group might depend on him. When faced with overwhelming problems, they consult the shaman, paying for his services with food, livestock, goods, or money. The problems cover a broad range: crimes, illnesses, bad luck, disasters affecting crops, and so forth. Shamans divine the whereabouts of missing persons and objects, identify the perpetrators of thefts and murders, find the reasons for misfortunes, and diagnose and treat disease. It is only this last activity that I will discuss in these pages. Shamanism is a vast subject, highly romanticized of late, and of great interest and appeal to Westerners. There are many good books on it as a way of viewing the world and as a practical attempt to control good and evil.[1]

The shamanistic conception of disease is different from that of orthodox medicine and from that of any of the alternative systems reviewed so far. Shamans attribute diseases to specific causes, just as allopaths do, but the causes they identify will seem very strange to conventional doctors. Witchcraft, demons, and malevolent supernatural forces are the major causes of medical problems in the shaman's world. Demons and evil spirits may enter human bodies, bringing ill health with them. Sorcerers and hostile shamans may entice souls from bodies, rendering people susceptible to harmful influences. They may also intrude objects of evil power, such as crystals, pebbles, or small animals, into victims by magical means, so that the objects cause suffering directly. Certain kinds of dreams may also bring on sickness, as may the violation of taboos or failure to perform required acts; such transgressions bring retaliation from gods and spirits.

In general, shamans do not believe in any natural sickness or death. They may admit natural agencies of illness but see them as secondary. A man may develop an infection from cutting himself with a dirty knife, but what made the knife slip? An evil thought might be the real cause, or a witch's curse. Some evil-working enemy is behind every medical calamity, and the shaman's job is to identify the evil power and neutralize it. This is just the way of thinking that Hippocrates tried to lay to rest when he ascribed all disease to natural causes and began to develop a science of rational treatment, but it remains alive and influential in much of the world. Shamans are as fascinated by (and as rigid about) black-magical causes of disease as allopaths are by germs.

In the course of investigating medicinal plants and unorthodox medicine, I have visited many shamans, mostly in South America. They have been a varied lot, ranging from drunks interested mainly in finding customers for hallucinogenic drugs to highly skilled practitioners who struck me as master psychotherapists. Some seemed genuinely able to promote healing.

One who impressed me favorably was a fifty-five-year-old Ingano Indian named Luis, who lived in a remote area of jungle in southwestern Colombia. He had practiced for twenty-two years and was an expert in the use of an Amazonian hallucinogenic drink called yagé (or *ayahuasca*), prepared from a woody vine (*Banisteriopsis caapi*) and the leaves of a related plant (*Diplopterys cabrerana*), both containing strong psychedelic drugs. Luis held yagé ceremonies every Saturday, cooking the beverage from scratch, then consuming it after sundown in an elaborate ritual with whoever turned up at his isolated hut. His reputation as a healer was growing when I visited him. Every Saturday, sick people made their way to him — not an easy journey. To get there I had to fly to the provincial capital, endure a torturous all-day bus ride to the end of the road system, travel a full day by river to a tiny and lawless port town, then walk three hours through jungle on a moderately difficult trail, all of this in an area of Colombia rife with guerrillas and soldiers. Some of the people who make this journey are really sick and have to be helped by friends or relatives. People come with bad infections, high fevers, convulsions, paralyses, and many other organic problems.

Luis treats them all, giving everyone doses of the hallucinogenic drink, even very young children, pregnant women, and those with high fevers. He consumes large doses himself and spends the entire night chanting, dancing, and praying in order to heighten his visions. He says the visions show him the causes and cures of sicknesses. In the morning he gives his diagnoses and recommendations, often prescribing medicinal plants he grows around his hut or collects from the forest. He also sees pharmaceutical drugs in his visions and tells some patients to buy particular ones as soon as they can get to a pharmacy. Luis is uneducated, with limited experience of the world beyond his remote home. He says he has learned most of what he knows from visions and from the spirit of yagé, including the uses of medicinal plants and pharmaceutical drugs.

My interviews with some of the patients convinced me that Luis had helped them, or, at least, that they felt they had been helped. Some described dramatic cures, and a few said Luis had made them better after regular doctors had failed. Assuming such reports are true — and I fear that a real obstacle to understanding shamanistic cures is the questionable accuracy of second- and thirdhand stories — what is Luis doing?

The drug he gives everyone certainly plays a role in his successes. Yagé is a strong emetic and purgative as well as a psychedelic; it cleans out the entire digestive tract in a spectacular fashion. Those who drink it know they have taken a real drug, not some inactive placebo.[2] Yagé also induces profound and strange states of consciousness, especially in the setting of the shaman's hut by night and candlelight and under the influence of his ceremonial performance. In these mental states, suggestibility increases, just as it does in hypnosis. Moreover, patients who come to Luis have invested considerable faith in the trip, braving physical hardships and dangers to reach him and confronting unknown and terrifying forces in his presence. All of these factors seem to me to favor therapeutic success.

Gastrointestinal purging cannot be bad for most sick people, certainly not in tropical regions, where intestinal parasites are universal. Those who fear shamans and mind-altering drugs are as likely to respond well to them as those who are positively attracted. Whether positive or negative, it is the strength of the emotional tie to the shaman that allows him to make a real impression on a client. Above all, Luis's long experience in the role makes him a powerful manipulator of the expectations and beliefs of those who come for help. On top of that, his prescriptions, whether of plants or manufactured drugs, may affect patients, too, both directly and indirectly by eliciting placebo responses. I doubt that I could ever sort out what did what in any clear-cut case of cure following one of Luis's ceremonies, but I am sure that belief is the key factor: the belief of patients in Luis's power as a healer, their hopes and fears of interaction with him, their expectation of cure, and the suggestions he gives them for interpreting the strange experiences they have in the ceremonies.

Some shamans use particular techniques of diagnosis and treatment to impress patients and hold their attention, such as rubbing eggs on the body, then breaking the shells and reading the nature of the disease in the patterns of their contents, or sucking the body to extract evil objects. The sucking method can be very dramatic, especially when the shaman vomits afterward, to expel the bad influences he has removed, or produces an actual object from his mouth, say a tuft of down covered with blood. Western doctors often sneer at this last manipulation as clever sleight of hand, used to fool credulous patients. Often, however, the patient knows the object was really in the shaman's mouth all along. That knowledge need not lessen the symbolic importance of the act or diminish its therapeutic power.

There is a documentary film called *Sucking Doctor* about a Pomo Indian shaman in California named Essie Parrish, who relied on this technique. She also used her hand to draw out disease. Anthropologists liked to study her because she was very open about her methods and so successful as a practitioner that sick people, Indians and non-Indians, came from far away to be treated by her. Here are some of her own words:

> When I work with the hand power it is just like when you cast for fish and the fish tug on your bait — it feels like it would with the fish pulling on your line — that's what it is like. The pain

sitting somewhere inside the person feels like it is pulling your hand towards itself — you can't miss it . . .

When I take it out you can't see it. You can't see it with your bare eyes, but I see it. Whenever I send it away, I see what the disease is. When the disease comes down into a person, which the white people talk about way different; and we Indians, we shamans, explain it way differently. That disease that comes down into a person is dirty; I suppose that is what the white people call "germs" but we Indian doctors call it "dirty" . . .

There is a doctoring power in my throat. Here somewhere in my throat the power sits . . . When I first doctored with my throat, it was for a young woman. When I treated her and sucked the disease out, something like a bubble came up out of my throat; just as it would if you blew up a big balloon, that is how it came from my mouth. Everyone there saw it. It had become inflated quite a lot when it floated from my mouth. Everyone saw it. Like foaming soap bubbles would look; that is how it looked at the start.

Ever since that happened I have been sucking diseases out . . .

That disease flies and sticks to a certain place in the mouth. Our [shamans'] teeth have the power; there is something attached to our teeth. There is where the power is, on one certain tooth. There is where the disease sticks. Sometimes it flies under the tongue. When it sticks there it is extremely hard to release . . . Then it dies there.

I spit out the dead disease. Then I let it fall into my hand so that many people can see it. They always see the disease that I suck out. But that is not to be touched by anyone else — it is contagious. Whoever picks the disease up, into him it would enter . . .

You can put it into something like a piece of paper or a basket. If you are going to do that, you should sing for that purpose, you should call for that purpose. Some diseases sit for a while — sit for a few minutes — but others are fast. Some fast diseases stay just for so many minutes after being put down and then disappear.[3]

Whatever one may think of Essie Parrish, it is clear that she has a strong, coherent system of belief about disease and its treatment and about her own healing work, validated by many consistent experiences.

Group healing ceremonies of high emotional charge are also common in shamanistic societies. Among some African tribes, masses of people may participate in healings that include days and nights of dancing, singing, and drumming. The Navajo of Arizona and New Mexico are famous for their "sings" — healing ceremonies that go on nonstop for a week or more. A sick person wanting a sing must pay for it. The fee can be considerable, and preparing for the event becomes the focus of the patient's life, requiring the full-time aid of family and friends.

Navajo medicine men treat illness by coordinating the sings but do not diagnose it. Diagnosis is the job of special individuals who go into trance to determine what is wrong but do not provide treatment. One variety of diagnostician is the hand trembler, whose hand, during trance, will begin to shake automatically and point to certain parts of the patient's body. These specialists are indispensable in Navajo society but do not have the power or prestige of the medicine men.

Navajo medicine men are symbolic healers rather than true shamans. They concern themselves with controlling good and evil and restoring harmony in the universe, the tribe, and the sick person, but they do so purely by manipulations of symbols, not by leaving their bodies, traveling to other worlds, or extracting psychic weapons. They rely on ritual, on very lengthy chants, and on the construction of symbolic patterns, using sacred objects, colored sand, and costumed dancers representing particular spirits. Hundreds of persons may attend these complex ceremonies, which are the main events of Navajo religion, bringing a tremendous power of shared belief to them. Many Navajo testify to their success in curing illness that resisted all other approaches.[4]

Among the Navajo, as in some other tribes that live in the midst of Western society, medicine men often recognize the value of scientific medicine and see no conflict between it and their traditional practice. They may even urge Indian patients to go to reservation hospitals for treatment of physical symptoms, because reduction of pain and discomfort will facilitate the more important job of restoring total harmony of body, mind, and spirit and putting back into its proper place the evil that caused disease to begin with. The white physician can treat superficial manifestations of illness in the body, while the nonwhite medicine man concentrates on its deeper roots and causes.

In anthropological accounts of shamans, reports of medical cures occur frequently, often in non-Indians, and sometimes with documentation.[5] Yet I am cautious about this kind of information in view of the present tendency to romanticize shamanism and the common desire to believe in magical cures.

I once attended a scientific meeting on human potentials that featured a performance by an Indian medicine man from Nevada. He attempted to heal the injured leg of a young man, quite swollen, discolored, and tender from a recent fall. The ceremony was long, dramatic, and moving. It included extensive sucking of the leg and vomiting into a bucket, in the midst of ritual purifications, prayers, and invocations of help from the Great Spirit. I happened to be sharing a room with the patient and had a good chance to examine his leg before and after the ceremony. I could not detect any objective improvement in appearance, tenderness, or mobility the next morning. Nor could the patient, although he reported that it felt "a little better" and that he was much affected by the ritual because he had never had anyone "pay that much attention to me."

Nonetheless, the assembled scientists all came to regard the medicine man's intervention as successful. Over the next few days, they talked up his powers more and more. Much later, a book appeared about the man.[6] It opened with a description of this incident, presenting the case as an example of significant objective healing not attributable to ordinary processes and remarkable by conventional medical standards.

I have no doubt that shamans cure people, but how frequently and of what conditions I do not know. I suspect they are most successful with what allopaths call "functional" and "psychosomatic" ailments but that they are occasionally able to cure serious organic disease as well. It is too bad that physicians pay so little attention to shamanistic treatment. Most studies are by anthropologists, psychiatrists, and psychologists, who are seldom skilled in physical diagnosis and the evaluation of organic disease.

Clearly, shamans work best for people who hold traditional beliefs in their powers, but, also clearly, they sometimes cure diseases in Western city dwellers who make long journeys to see them, often in desperation. Whatever their specific techniques, whether they operate individually or participate in large group ceremonies, give drugs or not, diagnose by visions or by reading eggs and entrails, suck out evil influences or travel to other worlds to capture straying souls, shamans make use of the power of belief — their own belief and that of their clients in the causation and moderation of illness.

Mind Cures

The pure healing power of belief, untrammeled with the paraphernalia of shamanism, is most evident in the persistence of systems of treatment best categorized as mind cures. The most famous example is Christian Science, but a number of parallel systems exist with similar origins and practices. Most came out of nineteenth-century America, nurtured by transcendentalism and full of optimism about the power of positive thinking and its potential to bring about self-improvement. Proponents of these systems were often women who were religious without adhering to any standard church or dogma. They believed that God was a source of pure goodness and unlimited power — power that became available to human beings who attuned their minds correctly to the divine reality. They also believed that matter was unreal or that it was less real than mind and totally subject to it.

Mary Baker Eddy (1821–1910), the founder of Christian Science, was the most persuasive champion of mind cure. She taught that disease, injury, pain, even death, are all illusions or mistaken thoughts, made apparently real and given power to influence behavior by minds out of harmony with God. Christian Science depends not on will power but on thought reform: restructuring beliefs to destroy these illusions at their source.

Mrs. Eddy was chronically ill for much of her early life. She sought help from homeopathy and magnetic healing (mesmerism); then, in 1866, following a severe accidental injury when her friends and relatives thought she was near death, she "discovered" the basic principle of Christian Science and rose from her bed, cured. Thereafter, she was able to initiate healing in others, sometimes just by visiting patients and spending a few minutes in prayer with them. Few of her followers were able to bring about dramatic cures in this way, but Mrs. Eddy began to teach a system of treatment designed to increase the healing abilities of her students.

Nine years after her own spontaneous cure, she published her monumental work, *Science and Health with Key to the Scriptures*. In it she wrote: "After a lengthy examination of my discovery and its demonstration in healing the sick, this fact became evident to me, — that Mind governs the body, not partially but wholly. I submitted my metaphysical system of treating disease to the broadest practical tests."[7] In 1879 she founded the first Christian Science church, reorganized in 1892 as the First Church of Christ, Scientist, with headquarters in Boston.

Perhaps because she had earlier been involved with mesmerism, Mrs. Eddy vigorously denied that her methods had anything to do with self-hypnosis or autosuggestion, but she talked a lot about suggestion. Ideas of pain and disease are bad suggestions that reinforce old illusions. The Christian Scientist should not study hygiene or anatomy, lest those studies add more detail to wrong ways of thinking about the body; nor should people record their ages, since that act gives reality to the concepts of aging and death. A woman I know, now in her forties, who was raised as a Christian Scientist, was forbidden to play doctor and nurse as a child: more bad suggestion. Reading ordinary newspapers is also bad — too much reinforcement of the illusions of injury, disease, pain, and death. Instead, one should assimilate wholesome thoughts that develop the innate power of the mind to transform physical reality and undo the appearance of negative manifestations. The best source of inspiration is *Science and Health*. Christian Scientists attribute many cures to the simple act of reading this book.

By devotion, study, and practice, Christian Scientists can develop the ability to heal themselves. They may also seek the professional services of special practitioners, who are licensed as healers by the Mother Church in Boston. The goal of Christian Science practice is to realize the illusory nature of one's ailments. Once the mind truly accepts that idea and experiences it as a reality, all afflictions of the body will melt away.

Christian Science treatment is a form of intensive prayer. Practitioners — mostly women — attempt to attune their minds to the all-encompassing goodness of Spirit, tap the infinite energy of that source, and direct it toward the sick to promote healing. They need not be physically present with their clients, because Christian Science treatment works at a distance. Many practitioners perform absent healing, having no more information than a client's name and telephone number and a sketchy idea of the problem. Licensed practitioners charge fees, just like other health professionals.

It is easy to lampoon the philosophy and methods of Christian Science. Mark Twain, for one, had a field day with it. In one sketch from 1903, he recounted his first visit to a practitioner, one Mrs. Fuller, following a fall that left him with a number of dislocations, fractures, and bruises. After instructing her client in the illusory nature of his injuries, Mrs. Fuller retired to perform absent healing on him, while the battered Twain sought more immediate relief from a horse doctor, who set his bones and charged a minimal fee. In Twain's words:

> Mrs. Fuller brought in an itemized bill for a crate of broken bones mended in two hundred and thirty-four places — one dollar per fracture.
> "Nothing exists but Mind?"
> "Nothing," she answered. "All else is substanceless, all else is imaginary."
> I gave her an imaginary check, and now she is suing me for substantial dollars. It looks inconsistent.[8]

Nevertheless, testimonials to the efficacy of Christian Science treatment are easy to find. The Mother Church began collecting them early on and has published many, some with medical documentation. Here is one account from a woman in Chicago:

> In November, 1907, it became necessary for me to have an upper tooth extracted. Owing to the diseased condition of the tooth and complications, the wall of the antrum was punctured and the jawbone splintered, resulting in the formation of an abscess and proud flesh.* One dentist insisted upon immediate treatment because the condition had become chronic. Another dentist, whom

---

*"Proud flesh" is an old term for a rare and unexplained complication of wound healing in which granulation tissue — the granular, red connective tissue that fills in wounds — proliferates abnormally, sometimes to the point of mushrooming out of the wound.

I had requested to examine the wound, informed me that the case was one for a competent dental surgeon and recommended an immediate operation.

The fragments of the truth that I had gathered from the study of the Christian Science textbook led me to seek the aid of a Christian Science practitioner, rather than trust my case to surgery, and the divine guidance in this way was fully demonstrated. The case was completely met in the first treatment, so far as the pain, etc. were concerned, and in a short time the wound was completely and perfectly healed. During the healing process, seven splinters of bone came out through the gum, without causing any pain. Later, I returned to consult the dentist who had recommended an operation, and after a careful examination, he assured me that the healing was perfect. He also told me that the operation in such a case would have been a difficult one to perform and was rarely successful.

[There follows a certifying letter from the dentist attesting to the cure and giving the findings of his examinations before and after the Christian Science treatment.][9]

Christian Scientists tend to be intelligent and educated, quiet and nonfanatic. They have engaged in interesting legal battles to preserve their right not to be treated by allopaths (as in refusing required immunizations) and must conscientiously resist the incorrect ways of thinking bombarding them every day from a world dominated by illusion.

Christian Scientists are found in many countries, but most live in North America and Europe, in those societies where public health is best. Even though they dismiss such possibilities as typhoid fever from contaminated water as unreal, they live among people who take them seriously and work to prevent them, as by chlorinating public drinking water. Christian Scientists would surely have a much harder time in the underdeveloped countries of the tropics.

When a Christian Scientist falls ill, the religion explains it as a lapse of vigilance over erring thoughts. Treatment must be directed to that sphere, but Mary Baker Eddy did allow some concessions to physical reality. She taught that it was all right to go to M.D.'s for purely mechanical problems — surgery, fractures, dislocations — and to take pain medication for them. She also permitted such general preventive measures as brushing teeth and wearing protective clothing, and even authorized taking time off from work or school and adopting a sick role while praying for a cure.

The lifestyles of Christian Scientists probably favor general health, since they tend not to drink, smoke, or engage in riotous living. Because they commonly intermarry with nonbelievers, family members often pressure them into going to doctors if they get really sick, and these visits may result in early detection and treatment of serious problems. Incidentally, allopathic doctors who have treated Christian Scientists consistently report that they are excellent patients, responding more quickly and favorably to drugs than others do. I find this piece of information most interesting. It has to do, I think, with Christian Scientists' fear of and fascination with regular medicine as the work of the Devil. By this negative belief they give it power.

Christian Science has survived the technological revolution of the twentieth century, and though it may be dwindling in numbers of adherents, there are still Christian Science churches and reading rooms in most American cities, the *Christian Science Monitor* still publishes its version of more wholesome news, the Mother Church keeps up its work, and practitioners treat the sick. Anyone interested in this distinctive system can easily find people who use it and can verify that real cures of real diseases regularly follow the purely mental and spiritual interventions of its practitioners, even in the midst of a society that thinks erroneously and despite the fact that at the age of eighty-nine Mary Baker Eddy, like all other human beings, succumbed to a most convincing illusion of death.

Faith Healing

Faith healing is as noisy and theatrical as Christian Science is quiet and reserved. In our society, faith healing is associated with Christianity, especially of the Fundamentalist sort, but practices like it occur in many parts of the world as rituals of many religions.

Christian faith healers take their inspiration from Biblical descriptions of healings performed by Jesus. The most explicit passage in the Bible is from James 5:14–16:

Is any sick among you? Let him call for the elders of the church; and let them pray over him, anointing him with oil in the name of the Lord: And the prayer of faith shall save the sick and the Lord shall raise him up; if he have committed sins, they shall be forgiven him.

Confess your faults one to another, and pray one for another, that ye may be healed. The effectual, fervent prayer of a righteous man availeth much.

Like proponents of mind cure, Christian faith healers rely entirely on belief to treat disease, but the philosophies of these two kinds of practitioners are distinct. The God of the faith healer is not an abstract, all-benevolent source of infinite power, waiting to be tapped by a properly attuned human mind. Rather, He is a personal deity demanding worship, who might refuse to respond to human requests for aid. For the faith healer, reality is not a unified realm of mind or spirit, but a vast battleground contested by God and Satan. Human beings are fallen and in need of redemption through suffering, not innocent victims of erroneous thinking. Pain, disease, and death are quite real, all part of God's plan. If attempts at healing fail, the practitioner of mind cure interprets the trouble as error and prescribes more effort to purify thought. The faith healer sees failures as the whim of an unpredictable deity or the just deserts of unworthy sinners.

Americans experience faith healers through direct participation in revival meetings, through newspaper accounts of miracle cures, and through radio and television programs. On the airwaves, popular evangelists loudly implore God and Jesus to heal the sufferers who come before them in front of large and enthusiastic audiences.

The tabloids are full of stories of religious healings. One recent article, headlined MIRACLE NUN FLOATS IN THE AIR AND HEALS THE INCURABLY ILL, credits an Italian nun with the ability to appear in several places at once, levitate, come to the faithful in visions that warn of danger, and heal the sick and dying. Another, titled MIRACLE OF THE JUNGLE SHRINE, describes a swampy lake in Cameroon, very difficult to reach, that began to heal people after a Roman Catholic priest blessed a rock near it and placed a statue of the Virgin Mary there. A blind villager suddenly regained his sight while bathing in the lake, and his story drew thousands of desperate people to the site. The article recounts the case of a middle-aged French nurse, blind for ten years as a result of diabetes, who made the arduous pilgrimage to the spot and was rewarded by getting her sight back as she emerged from the murky water.

There are innumerable accounts of this sort, and, again, the problem is credibility. Did the events really happen, or are the tabloids just catering to the wishful thinking of the average reader? Is there any medical documentation before and after the fact? If blindness was cured by a dip in an African pond, was it organic blindness due to retinal damage or functional blindness due to a conversion reaction — the province of the psychiatrist rather than the ophthalmologist? There is no way to know.

I have the same problem watching faith healers on television. When a crippled woman throws away her crutches and takes tentative steps after being pummeled in the name of Jesus and cheered by the studio audience, just what has happened? What was the nature of her ailment? Is her increased ability to move a true and lasting physical change or a temporary improvement due to a fever pitch of emotion? There is no way to know.

Psychotherapists have written at length about faith healing and even looked for correspondences between it and their own methods. They admit the reality of cures of functional illnesses by faith healers, pointing out that belief is the key factor and emotional excitement the chief technique responsible for any successes, but they cannot see how faith alone can cure an organic disease.

The most careful examinations of faith healing by medical scientists have focused on miracle shrines and the people who visit them. Perhaps the most famous of these sites is the grotto at Lourdes, France, a holy place of the Roman Catholic faith. There, in 1858, a peasant girl* saw visions of a beautiful woman, later revealed as the Queen of Heaven, who showed her a little spring. Since then, Lourdes has grown into a major tourist center, served by direct jet flights from many countries. It is officially sanctioned by the Roman Church as a miracle shrine. More than

*Marie Bernard Soubirous, Saint Bernadette, canonized in 1933.

two million pilgrims visit Lourdes each year, including about thirty thousand who are sick. Many of the sick come as a last resort, having exhausted all conventional remedies. Every day of the year major religious ceremonies and pageants take place at the shrine, including processions of tremendous aesthetic and emotional impact, during which the sick fulfill their mission by plunging into the icy spring.

Accounts of miracle cures at Lourdes are more reliable than others, because the Church subjects them to intense scrutiny and refuses to accept them as genuine unless they pass strict medical criteria. Since the shrine has been in existence, fewer than a hundred cases have passed the test. One expert on religious healing, Dr. Jerome Frank, an M.D. interested in the power of belief and its role in all forms of psychotherapy, comments in his book *Persuasion and Healing*: "The evidence that an occasional cure of advanced organic disease does occur at Lourdes is as strong as that for any other phenomenon accepted as true."[10]

Yet such cases are not very common, probably no more so than those occurring in Navajo sings, Christian Science practice, or nonreligious settings. Frank and other medical scientists who have investigated the patterns of events at Lourdes regard the emotional state of the pilgrims as the main factor predisposing a successful outcome. They point out that the decision to make the journey often becomes the central passion in a sick person's life, sweeping him or her out of hopeless despair into a whirlwind of preparation and activity, usually with the support of family, friends, and fellow parishioners of a local church. They note that chances of healing seem to correlate with the length and difficulty of the trip, a correlation that has been called the Lourdes phenomenon. Presumably, the longer and harder the trip, the greater is the investment of faith. No native of Lourdes has ever been cured there. Analysts also point out that most cures take place in the midst of the ceremonial processions to the grotto, at the very height of emotional excitement generated by the religious pageantry.

One hard-nosed English psychiatrist has written, "There is probably no stream in Britain which could not boast of as high a proportion of cures as the stream at Lourdes if patients came in the same numbers and in the same psychological state of expectant excitement."[11] In other words, these commentators all attribute any healings at Lourdes to the minds of the patients and not to any direct influence of the place, either natural or supernatural. They also point out that many physicians see cases of inexplicable cures that would be labeled miracles if they occurred at Lourdes. Spontaneous cures happen from time to time, even of severe organic disease. They do not restrict themselves to holy places.

When cures do occur at Lourdes, they are not instantaneous and not out of ordinary biological experience. Awareness of the initiation of healing may be immediate on emerging from the grotto, but the physical process takes time and makes use of familiar bodily mechanisms, such as tissue regeneration, where possible, and adaptation to loss. As Frank notes succinctly, "No one has regrown an amputated limb at Lourdes."[12]

It is difficult to test the proposition that the power of faith healing resides in the mind of the patient, but one experiment in the medical literature is worth describing.[13] The subjects of the experiment were three hospitalized patients, all women, all severely ill. The first had chronic gall bladder inflammation with stones; the second had not recovered from major abdominal surgery and was "practically a skeleton"; the third was dying of metastatic cancer.

The physician in charge first authorized a well-known local faith healer to attempt to cure the patients from a distance without their knowledge. Nothing happened. He then told the patients about the faith healer and, over several days, built up their expectations of his ability to help them. He told the women that the healer would attempt to cure them from a distance at a particular time. In fact, the healer was not working then. At the stated time, all three patients improved dramatically. The second was permanently cured. The cancer patient, whose body was swollen with retained fluid, quickly eliminated it and recovered sufficiently from severe anemia and general weakness to go home and take over her household duties; she had no further symptoms until her death. The gall bladder patient also lost her symptoms, went home, and remained free of problems for several years.

*

The occasional successes of shamans, practitioners of mind cure, and faith healers all demonstrate the power of belief to affect the body and modify or reverse illness. It is easy to think that a shaman or faith healer has some special power over illness (indeed, shamans encourage this idea), but an overview of mind-mediated healing suggests that one person cannot heal another any more than a muddy lake or icy stream can. It is a patient's belief in outside practitioners or miracle shrines that gives them any power over illness.

14

Psychic Healing

THOSE WHO BELIEVE in psychic healing claim it operates independently of patients' belief. They describe it as the ability of certain gifted individuals to diagnose and cure disease by extraordinary powers of mind, unrecognized by science, ungoverned by conventional physical laws, and not necessarily dependent on any divine intervention.

Psychic healing, like psychic phenomena in general, is a hot political topic, polarizing people into believers and scoffers. I find the antics of both groups difficult to take. On the one hand, champions of psychic healing are often totally credulous, easily falling under the spells of frauds, tricksters, and con artists — more practiced at wishful thinking than scientific inquiry. On the other hand, self-styled guardians of the faith of modern science see it as their responsibility to ridicule and disprove any extraordinary occurrence as a threat to reason and logic. They are as much wishful thinkers as their opposites, with an emotional need not to admit any elements of mystery, magic, or nonrationality into their models of reality.

I have no interest in entering into this imbroglio. My research on marijuana in the late 1960s convinced me that truth is not discernible when emotional involvements produce this kind of polarization. Also, my experience does not qualify me to discuss the matter in detail. I have no firsthand evidence of psychic healing and must rely on second- and thirdhand accounts. As in the case of faith healing, the credibility of those accounts is always questionable, since good medical documentation is usually lacking. I feel compelled to include some words on the subject in portraying the range of therapeutic systems, but I will keep them brief.

I am perfectly willing to be open-minded about the possibility of psychic healing. That it cannot be explained by current physical mechanisms does not bother me very much. The nature of reality, as indicated by contemporary physics, is so much stranger than any scientist would have thought a hundred years ago that I am sure models can be found to explain telepathy, psychokinesis, precognition, and all the rest in ways consistent with scientific theory.[1] My main question about psychic healing, if it exists, is how cleanly it can be separated from faith healing. In most reported cases, patients are fully aware that psychic healers are working on them. If cures result, it is impossible to know what to ascribe to the direct actions of the healer and what to the belief of the patient.

To give an idea of the nature of psychic healing, I will summarize the activities of two famous men, both with long records of cures attributed to extraordinary powers, both studied extensively by medical doctors, and both described in accessible, published accounts. One was primarily a psychic diagnostician, the other a psychic physician and surgeon.

Edgar Cayce (1877–1945) was a native of rural Kentucky who spent most of his life in Virginia Beach, Virginia.[2] A simple, sane, religious man, free of the aberrations of most professional psychics, he had a remarkable capacity for entering trance states and coming up with information not available to his conscious mind. This talent earned him the nickname the Sleeping Prophet.

In the course of his career, Cayce performed many thousands of "readings" for clients who sought his help. He would simply lie down, close his eyes, and speak, often in response to questions put to him by associates, who would record his responses. On waking, he had no memory of what he had said. Many of the readings concerned medical problems, which Cayce would diagnose and prescribe for, recommending special diets, massages, and medications. Since he was a sixth-grade dropout, these medical readings were all the more impressive for their accurate use of technical terms with which the waking Cayce was unfamiliar. His prescriptions were often for compound remedies that baffled pharmacists until they looked up the ingredients in old books and found that Cayce had given exact and sensible recipes. One doctor, a homeopath, tested Cayce's medical knowledge by questioning him in trance. He would ask questions like "What is the shortest muscle in the body?" and Cayce would reply, *"Levator labii superioris alaeque nasi* — in the upper lip." This man came to work with Cayce.

It made no difference to the sleeping Cayce whether a client was in the same room with him or at the other end of the continent. Sometimes, given nothing more than a name, he would produce a stream of information about the person's circumstances and health, together with medical recommendations — information later verified by independent observers. Many patients who consulted Cayce got better when they followed the advice he gave them, even those with serious chronic conditions given up as incurable by scientific doctors. These cures were not instantaneous or magical, just unusual in view of the source of the treatments. Records exist of most of the readings, as well as medical documentation of some of the cures that followed.

A number of medical doctors visited Cayce. Some used him to help with difficult cases, and after his death, some continued to treat patients according to his recommendations. In fact, several Cayce clinics still exist in this country, staffed by M.D.'s who find the readings work well as a therapeutic system.

The Sleeping Prophet did not just talk about health. He sometimes gave tips on the stock market or directions for finding oil. Though others made money from this information, he never did. Many readings concerned past lives of clients, since the sleeping Cayce took reincarnation as a fact. He also talked at great length about Atlantis and prophesied planetwide cataclysms for the final years of the twentieth century.

Much of this material sounds like hogwash. I, for one, do not expect California to fall into the sea by 1998, creating a new coast near Phoenix, Arizona. I find many of Cayce's metabolic and hormonal explanations of specific diseases to be garbled and fanciful, such as his assertion that multiple sclerosis is an imbalance of the endocrine glands due to deficiency of gold. Also, I think the Cayce phenomenon, whatever it was, left the world with his death. His followers and descendants, who have meticulously catalogued all of his utterances, and those doctors who now attempt to practice medicine by their guidance simply are not as convincing as the Sleeping Prophet himself.

I have visited the Cayce clinic in Phoenix and watched the

progress of several patients through it. The methods used there are more naturopathic than allopathic: applications of warm castor oil packs, massages with peanut oil, dietary regimens, and prescription of Cayce remedies. They are not likely to harm and certainly help some people, although they lack the power of trance readings from a prophet and do not produce cures as regularly as when the living, sleeping Cayce advised the same methods.

If the Cayce phenomenon was genuine — and the second-hand evidence is convincing in its abundance and detail — it argues for the reality of a collective unconscious as proposed by C. G. Jung: a storehouse of universal symbols, knowledge, and wisdom, closed to ordinary consciousness but accessible through the individual unconscious mind. In trance, as in other unusual mental states where attention shifts to the unconscious realm, information in that storehouse may become available. Edgar Cayce in trance had access to knowlege his ordinary mind did not contain, but even then, he could not transfer it to his waking consciousness. That he could perceive and diagnose at a distance and describe past and future events suggests that the collective unconscious may be independent of the ordinary restrictions of time and space. That the readings as a whole seem to be a mixed bag of fact and fancy suggests problems in transmitting material from the collective unconscious. Perhaps accurate information sometimes got tangled with ideas and associations in Cayce's own unconscious mind. Psychoanalysis, hypnosis, and other techniques of mental probing all reveal the individual unconscious to be a territory of chaos and confusion.

The Brazilian healer Ze Arigo, who died in an automobile accident in 1971 at the age of forty-nine, was a complete psychic doctor. His methods were more dramatic and more puzzling than those of Edgar Cayce.[3]

Uneducated and practically illiterate, Arigo became a leading medical practitioner in Brazil, seeing hundreds of patients a day toward the end of his life. He never charged for his services; he made his living by holding down ordinary jobs. Arigo attributed his powers to the presence of a voice inside his right ear, the voice of a spirit guide named Dr. Adolfo Fritz, a German physician who had died in the First World War. Dr. Fritz told him what to do, gave him all the medical information he needed, and guided him through the surgical procedures he performed routinely. Arigo's career as a healer began at age thirty-two, when the spirit of Dr. Fritz took up permanent residence in his body. That event followed a traumatic series of recurrent, vivid dreams about the doctor, accompanied by blinding headaches and persistent auditory hallucinations of Dr. Fritz's voice demanding that Arigo begin treating the sick.

In the years before his death, Arigo's practice assumed a standard pattern. He would sit at a table in a little clinic on a street corner in the town of Congonhas do Campo, where he lived. Patients filed past, and Arigo dealt with them one by one, spending little time on each case. Often, his whole interaction with a patient took less than a minute. He seemed to be able to diagnose on the spot, usually without asking any questions. His explanation was that Dr. Fritz told him what the problem was.

Some patients Arigo sent away, saying to them, "Your time has come; there is nothing I can do for you; God bless you." He sent others away for other reasons, telling some, "What you have is not serious; don't waste my time; go see your own doctor." A few others he recognized instantly as malingerers or investigators for the Brazilian Medical Association, which had worked out an uneasy truce with him.

Most patients Arigo treated, the treatment consisting of a prescription. He would scrawl his prescriptions on notepads, then pass them to an associate who typed them into legible orders that were honored by many Brazilian pharmacists. A number of medical doctors, including several from the United States, watched Arigo work and examined his patients and prescriptions. They reported that Arigo prescribed recognized pharmaceutical drugs in appropriate ways, that dosages and drug combinations were sometimes unconventional, and that some of the drugs were exceedingly obscure, being listed only in pharmacopeias of a few European countries and unknown to most physicians. How did an uneducated and semiliterate Brazilian peasant come up with the names and uses of all these pharmaceutical products? Arigo said the voice in his right ear dictated what to write. One researcher subjected Arigo to a number of medical and psychological tests but could find nothing unusual about his body or brain.

Finally, on some patients Arigo performed surgery — surgery of a most extraordinary sort. He never used sterile technique or anesthesia. He used whatever instruments were handy: pocket knives, scissors, kitchen knives, even some that were rusty and dull. He worked exceedingly fast, completing the procedures in seconds or minutes. He removed tumors, diseased organs, and cataracts, usually in broad daylight and in plain sight of observers, including medical doctors who cared to watch. The patients experienced no pain or strange sensations while he operated. Their wounds healed very fast, and most reported relief or cure of their complaints. Several investigators filmed Arigo's surgery.

I regret that I cannot give a firsthand account of this treatment. I was planning a trip to Brazil to see Arigo when he was killed. My interest in him was kindled by a friend, also an M.D., who had spent time with him and seemed to me to be a good observer and reliable witness. For the reader this information is secondhand, but the best of its kind. My friend reported standing inches from Arigo on a dozen occasions when the healer removed cataracts. He saw Arigo plunge the blade of a pocket knife directly into patients' eyes, saw the eyeballs pushed forward from the pressure of the knife, then saw the blade withdrawn with the opacified lens. The patients apparently felt nothing at all but experienced immediate improvements in vision.

There are accounts of psychic or instant surgery from various parts of the world, nearly all of them suspect. Most psychic surgeons are sleight-of-hand artists who perform at night, by candlelight, with much distraction, in conditions that defy careful observation or interpretation of perceptions. From the reports I have collected, Arigo appears to have been something else; but lacking direct evidence, I cannot be sure, and in any case, I have no ready explanation for his surgical skills.

Leaving these aside and considering his primary method — instant diagnosis and the writing of prescriptions for pharmaceutical drugs — I see much similarity between Arigo and Edgar Cayce. Both men received valid technical information from sources other than their conscious minds, and both recommended treatments that helped sick people who consulted them. Where that information came from is a good question, one that may go unanswered until a great deal more is known about the mind. As for the success of psychic medical prescriptions, whether for pharmaceutical drugs or strange compound remedies, the problem of analyzing it is the same as for ordinary medical prescriptions. Patients might have gotten better anyway. The drugs and remedies might have directly caused improvements by their pharmacological actions. Or they might have indirectly done so by evoking placebo responses because patients believed in them and the powers of the practitioners who prescribed them.

In the case of psychic healers such as Cayce and Arigo, whose reputations and unexplainable talents brought them immense fame, the beliefs of patients must have been factors in the outcomes of visits. I suspect many sick people who went to Virginia Beach and Congonhas do Campo were in states of expectant excitement not unlike those of pilgrims to Lourdes. If so, the role of belief in producing cures attributed to these men might have been considerable, regardless of where their diagnoses and recommendations came from, regardless of the direct effects of the medications they prescribed, and regardless of the ordinary or extraordinary nature of their actions.

I would love to know more about psychic surgery and instant diagnosis, about the supposed abilities of some people to hasten biochemical reactions in test tubes or to stimulate plant growth and animal healing by means of touch or projection of mental energy, but I am not optimistic about the chances of collecting good evidence about these phenomena until the present polarized situation resolves. Until then, only prejudiced believers will bother to take them seriously and set up experiments, and the only others who will pay attention to the results will be prejudiced scoffers, determined to expose all extraordinary occurrences as errors, hoaxes, or ordinary events in disguise.

15

Holistic Medicine

HOLISTIC MEDICINE is an informal collection of attitudes and practices, not a defined system of treatment. Like naturopaths, holistic doctors are an odd assortment of practitioners, disaffected with orthodox medicine and committed to alternatives they see as safer and better.

I do not like the word *holistic*. It is a stilted, synthetic word, a cumbersome way of saying "whole," especially obnoxious in the phrase *holistic health*. Also, the word has become a loaded term that pushes the emotional buttons of many people, particularly conservative allopaths, in much the same way as *natural* does. I even have in my files a newspaper clipping from 1980 reporting an investigation by a medical board in Manitoba, Canada, of an M.D. charged with "practicing holistic medicine."

The holistic medical movement began in the 1970s, mainly in California, as a reaction to the excesses and deficiencies of allopathy, much like the Popular Health Movement of the nineteenth century. Its promoters included many allopaths, especially younger ones who sensed the readiness of disgruntled patients to pay for alternative treatments. If there is any coherent philosophy to holistic medicine, it is that regular practice limits itself by paying attention only to the physical body and that good medicine must take account of whole persons, including their mental and spiritual dimensions. I could not agree more with this sentiment. I helped start a "holistic health" association in Tucson, have attended many conferences on the subject, and have championed the ideals of the movement in lecturing to audiences of allopathic doctors, students, and patients. Nevertheless, I have strongly mixed feelings about the holistic medicine I see practiced today.

What I like about it is its openness to other models of health and illness and its willingness to experiment. I know a number of holistically inclined M.D.'s who will try out botanical drugs, work in association with chiropractors and other "fringe" practitioners, study such techniques as acupuncture, and consider the possibility that psychic healing is a reality worth documenting. All of this is to the good. I am also delighted to meet M.D.'s who concentrate on health and its maintenance rather than on disease and its treatment. Hygeia has long deserved more devotion from the ranks of allopaths. To see M.D.'s emphasize nutrition and discourage medication is a remarkable and welcome change.

Having expressed these sympathies, I must recite my list of complaints about holistic medicine as I encounter it in America of the 1980s.

First, like naturopathy, the movement has no theoretical unity or coherence besides the very general philosophy mentioned above. All sorts of practices go on under the banner of holistic medicine, some of them quite bizarre.[1] Second, I am bothered by the uncritical acceptance of unorthodox methods by doctors who call themselves holistic. Medical practices are not sound just because they are unorthodox. (Nor are they bad just because orthodox allopaths happen to use them.)

An example of a technique whose ready acceptance disturbs me is a diagnostic procedure called applied kinesiology.[2] It dates from the mid-1960s and was used mostly by chiropractors until a number of holistic M.D.'s added it to their repertories. Applied kinesiology uses muscle resistance as an indicator of organ weakness and intolerance to foods and drugs. The practitioner might ask the patient to extend an arm and resist downward pressure. The test is repeated as the patient puts the other hand on and off different areas of the body or as substances such as salt, sugar, and various drugs are placed on the body. Decrease in resistance of the arm muscles is supposed to signal internal problems at those areas or prove the harmfulness for that patient of the substances tested.

Lacking sound experimental evidence on the validity of this method, I cannot make a definite judgment about it, but I can say that it looks to me very much like a suggestive phenomenon.

Often, the practitioner will communicate to the patient by subtle cues the belief that resistance should decrease at a particular moment. For example, the common idea among holistic doctors that white sugar is bad leads them to expect arm weakness when sugar is brought into a patient's field. This expectation may cause them to press in a different way on the extended arm when testing sugar. Sometimes the difference in manipulation is unconscious and not obvious, but sometimes it is quite gross and, I suspect, deliberate. Consciously or unconsciously, applied kinesiologists know how to push down patients' arms when they want to.

Possibly, the technique does reveal information about the body, but only careful experimentation can confirm or deny that. Until good experiments are done, the doctor who makes diagnoses and recommendations on the basis of applied kinesiology is proceeding most unscientifically. This kind of testing may be no more accurate than the hair-shaft analysis so favored by naturopaths. At least that is an objective test. Applied kinesiology looks more like a parlor trick, and its enthusiastic use by holistic practitioners shows how uncritical they can be in taking up methods whose main appeal is their unorthodox nature.

A frequent accompaniment of this predilection is a sort of sappy notion that health and medicine, after the holistic revolution, will be all sweetness and light. If people eat natural foods, take nice herbs, do yoga and meditate, and massage each other lovingly, they will never have to deal with the unpleasantness of serious disease or with therapeutic interventions that are not fun. I suppose that is an attractive fantasy, but I see no reason to believe in it. Disease, as I explained early on, is the manifestation of evil in the body, and evil is a reality, at least in the world of relative experience. Management of it always requires acknowledgment of its existence and sometimes requires suffering. Any doctor who excludes the hard, dark, painful side of reality from his or her model of health and medicine will be powerless to modify many conditions of disease.

The tendency of holistic practitioners to make therapy pleasant leads them to embrace methods so subtle that they have little effect on most patients. Bach flower remedies are homeopathic dilutions of harmless wildflowers, developed by an English physician, Edward Bach (1886–1936).[3] They are supposed to treat "unhealthy" moods, such as loneliness, despair, and uncertainty. They are certainly easy to take and possibly affect some sensitive individuals, but they simply lack therapeutic clout. In the same way, color therapy — shining light of particular hues on sick people — may well affect body energies in subtle ways, but I doubt that it will do very much for organic problems except in occasional patients. Yet I meet M.D.'s who endorse these treatments because they fit their preconceptions of what holistic therapy should be, which is, above all, pleasant.

A number of holistic medical organizations have come into existence, including an American Holistic Medical Association. These groups hold conferences and publish newsletters but seem to me stuck at that level of accomplishment. It is easy to put on holistic medical conferences. Keynote speakers deplore the horrors of regular medicine and praise the new movement. Lecturers describe the wonders of biofeedback, meditation, and homeopathy, while assorted practitioners demonstrate their methods of massage, bony manipulation, and diagnosis by applied kinesiology and iridology (reading the iris of the eye for information on all organs and problems).[4] Smoking is discouraged and natural foods are served.

Beyond this kind of activity, I see little concrete progress from holistic medical organizations. There is no trend to establish holistic clinics according to any standards or to conduct research on unorthodox practices in a careful way or to turn widespread dissatisfaction with allopathy into an effective alternative system of medicine based on sound principles and methods. Without such changes, any advances in holistic medicine will be the achievements of individual doctors who work out intelligent styles of diagnosis and treatment on their own, taking due account of the mental and spiritual aspects of patients but also paying due regard to scientific fact.

Two examples I have seen of holistic medicine in action represent the best and worst of it. So as to end on a positive note, I will begin with the worse case.

A few years ago I paid a visit to a hot-springs resort now operated as a healing center with stress on "holism." The owners and staff were young and given to belief in the value of vegetarianism, raw-food diets, fasting, cleansing enemas, psychic diagnosis and treatment, the use of herbs (including some illegal, psychoactive ones), and almost all unorthodox medical practices. They were vehemently opposed to regular medicine. Periodically, they organized healing festivals attended by various practitioners, including some holistic M.D.'s who shared their values. At other times they provided therapeutic services to clients who came to the resort seeking relief of ailments. During my visit, I happened to be the only physician on the premises. Despite my best intentions, I found myself in an adversary role, continually playing the part of spoilsport.

On the night of my arrival, a young man approached me and asked if I was a doctor. When I said yes, he began recounting a list of strange symptoms that had come on him when he woke up that morning and were still present. He was flushed and feverish, had a burning thirst and painfully dry mouth, could not focus his eyes on near objects, and also had to protect his eyes from light, because it hurt them. He said he felt "out of it" as well, in a kind of dreamlike state. I asked him if, by chance, he also had difficulty urinating. Yes, he said, he had great trouble initiating urination.

I then asked him if he had ingested anything unusual in the past twenty-four hours, because these symptoms are diagnostic of blockade of the parasympathetic nervous system, usually a toxic state due to drugs found in plants of the nightshade family. One of these plants, sacred datura (*Datura meteloides*) grew in abundance on the property; I had noted it on my drive in. He said, no, he had not taken any drugs or unusual foods, just several cups of a medicinal tea prepared the night before by one of the healers on the resort staff.

I suggested that datura leaves might somehow have found their way into the tea, but this brought an angry denial from the person who had made it, an intense young man. I asked him what was in the tea. He recited a short list of innocuous herbs — peppermint, chamomile, and the like — and said the mixture had the ability to purify the body.

A number of other guests who had listened to our conversation now came forward and admitted that they, too, had the same symptoms, though in lesser degree. All of them had drunk the same tea. As far as I could determine, everyone who drank it now had symptoms of nightshade poisoning, and no one had those symptoms who had not drunk it. The original patient then said that on the tea maker's urging, he had eaten the residue at the bottom of the teapot to "get all the benefit" from the brew. I reiterated my contention that the tea must have contained datura or some other nightshade drug.

Now I was shouted down and accused of being a "typical allopath." The brewer insisted that his tea was a powerful purifier. If people who drank it experienced strange symptoms, it was the result of toxins coming out of their livers under the influence of the tea — toxins that had accumulated during months and years of unhealthy living. The original patient, whose symptoms were most marked, must have had the worst build-up of toxins, and he should be happy they were now being eliminated by means of natural, herbal treatment. This explanation won out; mine was rejected as "narrow-minded."

That same night I watched someone else give a most unusual massage. He rubbed a patient's toes for such a long time that he abraded the skin on the upper surfaces, leaving large raw areas. The recipient of this treatment complained of the irritation but was silenced with the admonition that he should welcome the "stimulation" because it would improve energy flow around his body and so initiate healing of a number of minor ailments he hoped to lose.

The next morning, this hapless patient's toes were inflamed, showing signs of early infection. They were beginning to ooze a purulent fluid. Yet he sat contentedly, dangling his feet in a hot pool, while various practitioners and other patients congratulated him on the success of the treatment. Obviously, they said, his body was now discharging toxins through his toes, a healing phenomenon brought about by the massage. My recommendation that he disinfect and bandage his wounds was soundly rejected.

All of this was done in the name of holistic medicine.

At about the same time, I visited another healing center, a small clinic run by a middle-aged allopath, whose attendance at several holistic medical conferences had inspired him to change his practice. He was, above all, a good doctor, intelligent, educated, observant, intuitive, and experienced. Exposure to holistic philosophy had simply reinforced existing traits in him: an openness to alternative methods and a willingness to regard consciousness as an important determinant of health and illness. Though not trained as such, he was also a good psychotherapist, convinced that most disease had roots in the mind and able to provide receptive patients with counseling or referrals to other practitioners who might help them change their attitudes.

I spent two days with him, watching him work. He was especially good at sensing what kind of treatments would be best for particular cases and had no hesitations about using standard allopathic methods when he thought they were indicated. He had built up a local network of alternative practitioners to whom he referred selected patients. The referrals were mostly to an acupuncturist (trained in the traditional Chinese system), a biofeedback therapist, an osteopath (who used bony manipulation), and a clinical hypnotist. On his own he had learned shiatsu, a form of tension-relieving Japanese massage that uses firm pressure with fingers and thumbs. He gave shiatsu treatment routinely, thereby gaining the advantage of therapeutic touch with many patients.

In addition, he invited various healers to join him in the clinic and demonstrate their methods. If he liked what he saw, he sometimes asked them to stay on as co-workers. During my visit, a woman from Hawaii was with him who treated patients by laying-on of hands and used meditation and chanting to harmonize the rhythms of the body. She told me she found these techniques generally helpful but added that her teacher in Hawaii maintained that "real healing can only take place through a change in consciousness; everything else is just therapy."

One patient at the clinic was a middle-aged woman just out of the hospital after surgery and radiation for a recently discovered uterine cancer. The doctor felt her primary problem had been controlled. His concern now was for her general health and comfort. The radiation treatment had been especially hard on her, leaving her weak and in pain. His recommendations included unconventionally high doses of vitamin A, a diet high in raw fruits and vegetables, regular use of an herbal tea widely valued in Mexico as an anticancer agent, and a program of meditation and visualization on her pelvis to speed healing. He regarded these treatments as complementary to the surgery and radiation he had also recommended when the tumor was first detected.

Another patient was a middle-aged man, a business executive with high blood pressure and early signs of coronary artery disease. The doctor had seen him before, reviewed his medical history, done a thorough physical examination, and ordered a few laboratory tests. He now gave his recommendations: a vegetarian diet (he arranged for the patient and his wife to take cooking lessons from the staff of a local vegetarian restaurant), a course of biofeedback training to lower blood pressure and promote general relaxation, a program of yoga exercises and meditation, and a graduated program of exercise.

Both patients have responded well to the regimens.

This physician calls himself a holistic medical doctor. Most patients who seek him out want something other than ordinary allopathic treatment without taking their chances on practitioners too far from the scientific mainstream. His mixture of originality, unconventionality, and good medical judgment inspires confidence and belief, and, in my estimation, brings great credit to the name of holistic medicine.

16

Quackery

QUACK is a wonderful word, pithy and sharp, the perfect insult for disliked medical practitioners of all persuasions. Its origins are not obvious. Some people think it is the same *quack* that a duck makes, because snake-oil salesmen hawk their wares in loud, persistent tones resembling the noise of that animal. Actually, the word is a short form of *quacksalver*, the Dutch equivalent, with the literal meaning of "a user of gooey ointments." *Quacksalver* is built of two Germanic roots, one of which surfaces in our word *salve*, the other in *quagmire*. It is the latter, suggesting sliminess, that comes down to us as the medical quack.

Quacks keep company with such other colorful characters as mountebanks and charlatans. The mountebank steps up on a platform, as his name suggests, in order to toot his horn. *Charlatan* is a French word from Italian *ciarlatano*, variant of *cerretano*, designating an inhabitant of Cerreto, a village in central Italy said to be famous for its quacks. I would love to know more about Cerreto and its people and hope an international conference on unorthodox treatment will one day be held there.

If the etymology of *quack* is obscure, its definition is difficult. My dictionary says that a quack is an untrained person who pretends to have medical knowledge, but what is training and what is medical knowledge in view of the diversity of systems of treatment? Any new or exotic therapy will be quackery to the orthodox until it establishes itself. Homeopaths were quacks in the 1700s and 1800s until they obtained better cure rates for epidemic diseases than allopaths did. Osteopaths were quacks in the days of Andrew Taylor Still. Most allopaths still regard all chiropractors as quacks, and before the 1970s, they would surely have put in the same category any doctor who used acupuncture. Besides, if belief is an important key to healing, even methods based on wrong assumptions and methods devoid of significant effects of their own may elicit real cures by means of the placebo response.

Nevertheless, there is real quackery in the world. I may not be able to define it simply, but as with pornography, I know it when I see it. Here is a clear example from an earlier era:

In 1892 one Dr. Hercules Sanche of New York City obtained a patent on a device called the Electropoise. He said it forced oxygen through the body. The Electropoise was a metal cylinder three and a half inches long, weighing five ounces and sealed at both ends. An uninsulated, flexible cord was attached to one end. At the free end of this cord was a small disk meant to be fastened to the patient's wrist or ankle by an elastic band. The Electropoise was on the market by 1893. It sold for ten dollars. When investigators broke into the cylinder, they found it to be empty.

Soon after, Dr. Sanche applied for a new patent on an improved version called the Oxydonor, which, he said, "causes the human organism to thirst for and absorb oxygen, the vitalizer of the blood, through the myriad pores in the skin." In the Oxydonor, the cylinder was shorter and now contained a stick of carbon. It cost thirty-five dollars. To use it, you placed the cylinder in a bowl of plain water, attached the disk to your ankle or wrist, then relaxed. Sanche claimed the Oxydonor would "cure all fevers, including yellow fever, in a few hours" and also would "cure all forms of disease."

The Oxydonor was widely advertised in national magazines of the early 1900s. The advertisements showed a beautiful female model reclining on a sofa, reading a novel, with the disk attached to her ankle, her myriad pores presumably absorbing vital oxygen. This product was so successful that it inspired many imitations, including an Oxygenor King, an Oxytonor, a Duplex Oxygenator (with double cords and disks for *both* ankle and wrist), an Oxypathor, and an Oxybon. All looked similar, but the contents of the cylinders varied.

In 1915, Dr. Sanche was prosecuted for mail fraud.[1]

I do not know whether Hercules Sanche was a real doctor or

had any medical knowledge. Even if he did, it is reasonable to assume that his inventions were intended to deceive a gullible public and enrich his own coffers. I consider deception the essential element of quackery, as the dictionary suggests in defining a quack as an untrained person who *pretends* to have medical knowledge. Quacks love to trot out strange degrees and display ornate diplomas from bogus institutions. One I met in southern California called himself a Doctor of Healthology.

Quacks are found in all parts of the world. In my files is an article about Zulu witch doctors in South Africa. It quotes one Credo Mutwa, described as the "pope" of all the witch doctors in that country. He says, "All I need do is look at a patient to determine his trouble. If a witch doctor can't do that he is a quack. Unfortunately, we have many of those."[2]

Because health and disease play on powerful hopes and fears, and because many people want to avoid work and discomfort, medicine is a field made to order for charlatans. Scientific doctors unwittingly help quacks when they mystify patients rather than educate them about medical matters. People who understand the basic principles of health, healing, and treatment are not likely to fall for swindles like the Oxydonor or other health aids that use the trappings of technology to part customers from their dollars.

Practitioners who genuinely believe in their methods and who are able to create belief in patients about the possibility of cure are not quacks in my judgment, even if those methods are unorthodox and even if they turn out to be intrinsically worthless in scientific terms. Such practitioners may be able to function as effective therapists in spite of their methods.

The power of belief to yield good results even when ineffective practices elicit it is a favorite literary theme. Consider the Wizard of Oz, the good-hearted mountebank who appears in the classic American fable of the same name. His representations to be an all-powerful wizard are pure hokum, but, by believing in him, Dorothy and her friends not only accomplish tasks they never would otherwise think themselves capable of, they also get all their wishes and, in the end, realize it is their own powers that serve them, not any external agencies.[3]

Examples of the Wizard-of-Oz phenomenon abound in medicine. Healing is an innate capacity of the mind-body, waiting to be released or unblocked but not usually under voluntary control. Sick people often have to go to practitioners for healing to happen, and their belief in those practitioners may be more important than the direct effects, if any, of treatments. This conclusion is obvious from reviews of real cures that follow therapeutic interventions devoid of intrinsic efficacy.

Even quacks can produce the Wizard-of-Oz phenomenon in credulous patients, but their own knowledge of the worthlessness of their methods and awareness on some level that they are cheating people make them much less likely to create the kind of belief that favors healing. A believing practitioner's faith in a system of treatment can excite a patient's belief, and, combined, the two can accomplish miracles. Quacks can never do that as well as genuine doctors.

17

What Do All These Therapeutic Systems Have in Common?

I BEGAN STUDYING alternative medicine in 1970. Since then I have visited many practitioners of many different therapeutic systems, observing them at work, submitting myself to treatment as a patient whenever possible, interviewing other patients, and reading the works of the inventors of the methods. I have described some of the systems I have looked at. Even this partial selection constitutes a bewildering array. Now, as a neutral observer, unattached to any one practice, I will attempt to summarize my studies by listing six conclusions.

1. No System of Treatment Has a Monopoly on Cures

Every system I have examined cures some of the people some of the time. However strange, confused, or inconsistent with scientific fact, all formal therapies produce some cures. Scientific doctors may like to believe that the more bizarre ones — such as shamanism, faith healing, and Chinese medicine — work mainly in cases of functional illness, but every system I have examined, including those, can boast some clear cures of advanced organic disease. The frequency of such cures is unknown, because no research exists on the question, and it would be very difficult to collect the data. My impression is that dramatic, clear-cut cures of advanced organic disease following applications of medical treatments are not very common in any school of therapy, allopathic medicine included.

2. No System of Treatment Has a Monopoly on Failures

Every system I have examined fails to work some of the time, regardless of how logical and scientifically sound its theory, how careful its application, and how strong its indication for a particular problem or patient. Again, the frequency of failures is not known, but in my experience it is considerable for all systems, allopathy included.

The question of why treatments fail, when theory and experience predict success, is as important as the question of why treatments work when science can demonstrate their theories to be fallacious.

3. There Is Great Inconsistency Among Existing Systems of Treatment

In both theory and practice, rival systems of medicine are often irreconcilable. Homeopathic theory accuses allopathic medicine of creating chronic disease by suppressing superficial symptoms. Allopathic theory cannot find any reason why homeopathic remedies should work except by evoking placebo responses, but homeopaths reject that explanation. Scientific understanding of infectious disease provides no possible mechanism for the success of osteopathic manipulation in treating such conditions. Shamanism would predict acupuncture to be ineffective in treating illness because it does not address psychic causes, such as the presence of objects of evil power. No system can explain the actions of a psychic surgeon like Arigo.

The existence and success of therapeutic systems based on mutually inconsistent theories and methods must be accounted for by any general theory of health and healing. It suggests that factors other than theories and methods determine whether medical interventions succeed or fail.

4. New Systems of Treatment Work Best When They First Appear

One clear pattern in the material I have presented is declining power of new forms of practice over time. An inspired medical heretic and prophet is often able to produce dramatic cures of many kinds of illness. Samuel Hahnemann, Andrew Taylor Still, Mary Baker Eddy, and Edgar Cayce all could. These people may be able to communicate their skills to one or two generations of students, but over time, and especially after their deaths, the overall efficacy of their systems declines, even though the same methods remain in use, applied according to the master's directions.

5. Belief Alone Can Elicit Medical Cures

Cures of organic illness following visits to miracle shrines, faith healers, and Christian Science practitioners demonstrate that belief alone, without any physical intervention, is enough to bring about therapeutic success. This fact must also be included in any comprehensive theory of health, healing, and the role of treatment.

6. Belief in Treatment Is a Unifying Variable That Ties Together the Five Previous Conclusions

Belief in a system of treatment varies from practitioner to practitioner and patient to patient. Such variation can explain why any system works some times and not others. Since belief alone can elicit healing, the occasional success of treatments based on absurd theories is not mysterious. Since belief in a new system is greatest in its inventor and those in direct contact with that person, the declining efficacy of a system over time is also understandable.

Given the importance of belief as the crucial factor determining the outcome of treatment, it is necessary to look closely at the role of belief in the general context of mind-body interactions. By understanding the indirect relationship between treatment and healing, people will be able to take more responsibility for their own bodies and be better prepared to make intelligent choices of treatments and practitioners when they decide to seek outside help.

V

MIND AND BODY

18

Why Warts Fall Off

MIRACULOUS CURES of cutaneous warts are as commonplace as they are curious. Ask about them in any group of people, and you will easily collect typical stories. Usually, the warts were on the hands, most often in childhood or adolescence. The methods used to get rid of them range from the straightforward to the outright peculiar, with no consistency. For the past few years I have compiled a list of these methods. It is long and continues to grow. I defy anyone to show me what they have in common other than people's belief in them.

Techniques that have treated warts successfully include: being touched by a neighborhood wart healer, applying some curative plant to the wart, rubbing the wart with a cut potato and burying the potato under a particular kind of tree during a particular phase of the moon, selling the wart to a sibling by striking a bargain and exchanging money, handling some kind of animal. I hear about some of these techniques often, about others very rarely. One that came up only once caught my attention because it had nothing to do with the actual wart: a man I met at a conference told me that when he was a boy, his mother urged him to sneak down to the kitchen at night while she was asleep and steal something from the refrigerator; if no one found out what he took, his wart would go away, she promised. It did.

If there is no consistency to these procedures, there is great consistency in the response. Typically, a person will follow one of these suggested treatments in the afternoon or evening, then go to bed. Next morning, when the wart is touched, it sloughs off, leaving clean, pink skin. It does not regrow. A variant response is gradual shriveling and disappearance of the wart over the next week or two. Very many persons have experienced these dramatic cures in response to very many treatments having nothing in common except that people believe they will work.

Cutaneous warts are not functional problems. They are real, discrete, physical, organic growths, made up of abnormal tissue infected with viruses. Nevertheless, they are susceptible to virtually instant healing brought about by belief in treatments that cannot have significant direct effects on the viruses or the abnormal tissue.

Compared to the clear and lasting success of folk remedies for warts, the scientific approach of conventional medicine is pitiful. Allopaths attempt to deal with warts by cutting them off with knives, burning them off with electric sparks, freezing them off with liquid nitrogen, and etching them off with an acid so corrosive that great care must be taken to prevent its touching the surrounding skin. Not only are these methods crude, painful, and potentially mutilating, they are frequently ineffective. At least half the time, the warts grow back, often in multiple clusters.

It is revealing of the limitations of materialistic science that no serious research exists on wart cures in response to treatments based on belief. I can think of few medical phenomena more deserving of study. When a wart that has persisted for months or years falls off within hours of being rubbed by a cut potato, the cure may look miraculous, but it is not mystical. Some analyzable, physical mechanism must underlie the event, one that uses familiar body components such as nerves and blood. It would be valuable to identify and understand that mechanism, because it is powerful, precise, and efficient, able to reject diseased tissue (and prevent recurrence) within almost no time of being activated. Think of the possibility of directing that mechanism against malignant tumors or obstructions in coronary arteries or calcium deposits in joints! The prevalence of wart cures argues that the mechanism exists in everyone. Clearly, the switch that turns it on is located in the mind.

Of course, this last fact puts the phenomenon beyond the reach of most medical scientists. Because belief and the mind are immaterial, they appear invisible, unreal, or unimportant to the materialist. The obvious physical fact of wart cures is undeniable, but because its causal roots are in the nonmaterial realm, most doctors ignore it, fail to see its momentous relevance to medicine, and even treat it as a kind of joke. When I talk about wart cures with allopaths and biologists, they often recount their own favorite wart stories with smiles and laughter, as if these were nothing more than sources of entertainment.

Not taking wart cures seriously is the commonest recourse of scientists who realize that their model cannot explain these common events but who are not willing to admit the theoretical challenge they pose. Wart cures are a large, ugly anomaly for allopaths, explainable only by granting the tremendous importance of nonphysical factors in shaping the physical body. When confronted by them, many doctors will acknowledge their existence but refuse to admit their significance. Wart cures are just silly curiosities that make good stories, often told at the expense of patients, since they show how gullible patients can be. (Imagine, falling for that old cut-potato business!) I have presented my ideas on wart cures to many groups of medical doctors but have not had one of them ask, "How can we investigate this phenomenon and make use of it?" Instead, I have often had grinning physicians afterward say, "I've got a great wart story for you."

One doctor told me he had once treated a man in his late fifties who had lived for years with cutaneous warts over most of his body. The standard methods of removing them had only multiplied their numbers. Finally, on a whim, the doctor told the patient he would try out a new, experimental form of radiation that was somewhat risky but so powerful that it might knock out the problem. He and a radiologist colleague had the man remove his clothes and stand in a darkened X-ray room. Then they made the machines hum loudly without actually emitting any X-rays. The next day, all of the warts fell off. They did not grow back. The doctor was impressed, but it never occurred to him to try to find out what went on in the patient's mind-body or to consider the implications of what he had seen.

Occasionally, I meet doctors who make practical use of the mechanism even though they pay it no serious attention. I know of one dermatologist who keeps a lizard skull in a drawer of his desk. When discussing treatment for warts with certain patients, he produces this strange object and says, "I don't know why it is, but some people who come to me with problems like yours find their warts go away if they place their hand on this skull. Perhaps you would like to try that before you let me burn you." One man, who was taken to this doctor as a teenager, tried the lizard skull (to the horror of his mother) and was rewarded by the shrinking and complete disappearance of his warts within ten days.

In the absence of scientific studies of wart cures, I can only speculate about the nature of the mechanism. Clearly, the nervous system is involved, because belief has to be carried from the mind to the site of the wart by nerves. Possibly the circulatory system plays a role, perhaps by shutting off blood flow to the wart and weakening it. The immune system is another likely participant, since it includes specialized cells that can attack and destroy foreign matter and remove diseased tissue.

Warts may be especially vulnerable to this process because they are superficial and clearly demarcated from normal tissue. Also, they often disappear spontaneously without any attempt to influence them. Nevertheless, the mechanism responsible can be activated by belief and can resolve more difficult problems.

Warts on the sole of the foot are much more stubborn than warts on the hands. Plantar warts persist longer, regularly grow back and multiply after allopaths destroy them, and resolve spontaneously much less frequently. Still, I have seen them bend to the power of healing initiated by the mind. One plantar wart sufferer, a man in his mid-twenties, came up to me after a lecture and asked how he could make his wart go away. It had a long history, including multiple regrowth after allopathic incineration, now was very large, and often became painfully inflamed (a frequent occurrence with these growths, because their location exposes them to constant pressure).

I did not tell this man that plantar warts are harder to deal with than others. I did tell him that many methods were available to him; he needed only to pick one that appealed to him. He pressed me for a specific technique. On an intuitive impulse I told him to try rubbing the wart with a piece of dry ice before going to sleep one night. Then I asked him if he was a good visualizer. He said yes. I suggested that each night and morning he spend a few minutes in bed visualizing white light flowing from his head to his foot along a specific route, keeping in mind the idea that this light would help his body eliminate the wart.

Six months later, I got a letter from the man with a detailed story of what had happened. His talk with me had made him uneasy because it made him feel responsible for his wart. He could not find a source of dry ice, so did nothing for several weeks except become more and more guilty about not tackling the job. Finally, exasperated, he followed my advice with ordinary ice and began to practice the visual exercise. After a week, he could notice a change in the wart — it was slightly smaller. Elated, he continued his efforts, and the shrinking accelerated. After a month, the wart was gone for good.

Flushed with success, this man turned his white light on another problem: a ganglion on one wrist. Ganglions are benign tumors of tendon sheaths that can grow slowly to golf-ball size and often become inflamed and sore, limiting motion of joints. Conventional treatments are not very satisfactory. Country doctors sometimes used to smash ganglions with heavy Bibles, driving them out of sight, if not out of mind. Cortisone injections into the tumor suppress inflammation and relieve symptoms but do not change the physical structure of the growth. Removal is very difficult, because these tumors have complex attachments to tendons that make dissection a surgical nightmare.

Had this patient asked me about the likelihood of eliminating a ganglion by visualizing white light going to it, I would not have encouraged him. Unlike warts, ganglions are solidly walled off from normal tissue, indolent, and unlikely to go away spontaneously. Fortunately, I was not around to convey this pessimistic view. The man got rid of his ganglion with two months of regular visualization. Apparently, his body resorbed the tumor in its entirety. This case suggests that the mechanism underlying wart cures can work to heal other abnormal growths.

I can think of several ways to begin investigating that mechanism. A first step would be to record careful observations of the phenomenon, using warts on hands treated by hypnotic suggestion or some other single method. Since the most interesting response is complete rejection of the wart in a matter of hours, continuous observation of subjects would not be difficult. It might be worth monitoring temperature of the surrounding skin and blood flow in a finger. It might be worth looking for antibodies or other circulating factors in the blood at the time of a wart cure that would stimulate rejection of warts in other people.

My reasons for stressing the mechanism of wart cures are several. First, it is the objective, researchable aspect of the problem. Once its components come to light, doctors will be able to see the reality and importance of this example of mind-mediated healing. Second, the same mechanism may underlie other mind-body events, such as placebo responses, faith healings, spontaneous remissions of cancer, and so forth. Third, it may provide a key to elucidating the ways that mind and body impinge on each other. Fourth, understanding the mechanism of wart cures may enable people to activate it voluntarily in themselves or others and direct it toward more serious medical problems.

Cancer is an obvious possibility. It kills so frequently because the body seldom realizes that malignant tumors are abnormal and should be destroyed. Allopaths treat cancers much as they treat warts: they attempt to remove them by cutting, burning, or chemical attack, and their results are equally unimpressive. There is growing recognition that the surest way to cure cancer would be to get the immune system to recognize it and launch search-and-destroy missions against malignant cells. It is quite possible that the body can get rid of even large masses of cancerous tissue as easily as it can separate itself from a cutaneous wart, perhaps by the same mechanism. Documented cases exist of spontaneous remissions of most forms of cancer. In some of these, large tumors have disappeared within hours or days. If I were in charge of dispensing government funds for cancer research, I would certainly allot a large portion of them to studies of the mechanism of wart cures.*

I have been building a case for belief as the crucial factor determining the success or failure of medical treatments. Any treatment — whether allopathic drugs and surgery, homeopathic remedies, chiropractic manipulations, shamanistic rituals, or

---

*Warts and cancer may be related in origin as well as cure. The human papillomavirus (HPV), which is associated with warts, also is associated with cancer of the cervix and vulva in women and some skin cancers in both sexes.

Chinese acupuncture — includes two distinct elements: the direct effect of the treatment itself (if any) and the belief it elicits in both practitioner and patient.

Some treatments, such as allopathic drugs and surgery, obviously influence patients directly, although a cause-and-effect relationship between their use and any subsequent improvement may be anything but obvious. Internal mammary artery ligation as a treatment for angina pectoris certainly affects the mind-body strongly, but reduction in heart pain after the operation turns out to be reproducible by sham surgery with the artery left untied. For other treatments, such as homeopathic prescriptions and acupuncture, the direct effects, if they exist, are quite obscure and unexplainable in terms of known physical mechanisms. For still others, such as rubbing cut potatoes on warts, direct effects may exist, but it is reasonable to assume they are minimal and irrelevant. I do not think it would be worth performing exhaustive chemical analyses of potatoes in the hope of discovering some natural anti-wart factor.

The last category of treatments — those devoid of significant or relevant intrinsic effects — are known to doctors as placebos. Their power to cure is credited to patients' belief in them. The nature of placebos and the responses they can evoke interest me greatly, because they provide much more information about the complexities of mind-body interactions and their potential importance in medicine. Although doctors are very familiar with them, they commonly misunderstand placebos and fail to make full use of them, both in the theory and practice of medicine.

The wart cure is one example of a placebo response. It is also proof positive of the existence of innate healing ability — an ability so effective as to make most external therapeutic interventions look quite clumsy and feeble. This discussion of mind and body began with words and questions about wart cures because these cures are everywhere to be seen — not extraordinary occurrences like faith healings but the commonplace experiences of a sizable fraction, perhaps 50 percent, of the population. They are also utterly dramatic and, once you see them for what they are, totally convincing of the fact that belief is the master key to healing, that the physical mechanisms of cures of disease, whatever their nature, make connections to the immaterial realm of mind.

19

The Placebo Response

THE WORD *placebo* is Latin, meaning "I will please." It entered English first as a Roman Catholic Church word designating a particular vesper service, came to mean "flattery" and "flatterer," then found a home in the technical vocabulary of physicians. An 1811 edition of one medical dictionary identified it as "an epithet given to any medicine adapted more to please than benefit the patient."[1]

The strict definition of a placebo is an inert substance — a sugar pill — designed to look like a real drug and given to satisfy the desire of a patient for medicine when no indication exists for a genuine prescription. In discussing the extreme reliance of allopathic physicians on drugs to treat disease, I wrote that a patient who does not receive a prescription in the course of a visit to a doctor is likely to be disappointed, so pervasive is belief in materia medica and so universal the desire to take medicine. *Homo medicus* has been suggested as a better name for the human species than *Homo sapiens*, because that desire, more than wisdom, seems to be a distinguishing human characteristic.

When patients press doctors to satisfy their need to be medicated but present no objective signs of specific disease, doctors have several choices. They can give nothing, but then run the risk of losing patients. They can also give nonspecific medications to make patients feel better. The most effective drugs for this purpose are those affecting mood: alcohol, opium, and cocaine in the old days, amphetamines and tranquilizers more recently. The risk of this course is dependence. Psychoactive drugs often make patients feel temporarily high and forgetful of their ailments, but because the drugs do not affect underlying conditions, they lend themselves to repetitive use, and all can be habit-forming. Doctors who reject these alternatives have one other option: the placebo. It may send patients away satisfied, without causing any harm.

When physicians hand out placebos, patients often report improvement or disappearance of symptoms. Sometimes, objective signs of disease diminish with placebo treatment, and sometimes complete cures occur. These satisfactory results of treatment with substances devoid of intrinsic actions are usually called "placebo effects," but that term is inaccurate. Such results are not effects of the dummy pills but responses of patients to taking them. They should be called "placebo responses," and I will use that term.

Scientific interest in placebo responses has been very slow to develop. Not until 1945 did the word *placebo* appear in the title of a medical journal article.[2] Two reasons account for this, one practical, one theoretical. For many doctors, the practice of placebo medicine has an unsavory scent about it. It seems to involve deception and trickery and so is not clearly distinguishable from quackery. Many doctors never use placebos. Even those who do are often ambivalent about them, preferring not to discuss their use and certainly not their importance. A recent study on the use of placebos for pain relief in a university teaching hospital revealed some noteworthy patterns.[3] Doctors and nurses tended to give placebos to disliked patients they suspected of exaggerating their pain or to patients who did not respond to the usual medications. If the patients reported relief from the placebos, doctors interpreted their favorable responses as evidence that the pain had no physiological basis.

The theoretical obstacle to scientific research in this area is the same one I described in chapter 18 in writing about wart cures. Placebo responses originate in the mind, which seems to put them beyond the reach of scientific inquiry, at least to scientists dogmatically attached to the materialistic model.

Instead of paying enthusiastic attention to the placebo response as a major clue to the interworkings of mind and body and as a potential key to activating true healing, most doctors and researchers regard it as a nuisance, as something to be screened out or eliminated when testing new therapies. The most common usage of the word *placebo* I encounter in medical settings is in comments like "How do you know that's not just a placebo effect?" or "We have to rule out the placebo effect."

The only fully sanctioned use of the placebo is as a standard of comparison in evaluating new drugs, especially in double-blind tests, where neither patients nor doctors know who gets the real drugs and who gets the placebos until the tests end and all data are in. Drug researchers are very pleased with themselves at having come up with this method. (It dates back only to the 1930s and was not in general use till the late 1940s.) One medical writer, in commenting on the controlled evaluation of new drugs, gushes, "Twentieth-century medicine has merely refined the procedure to a nearly flawless level of efficiency."[4] Contemporary researchers think that the double-blind method absolutely screens out the contaminating influence of belief, so that if a new drug works no better than a dummy pill in this procedure, the drug may be confidently discarded as worthless, any apparent efficacy being "nothing but a placebo effect."

The inclination of physicians and researchers to assign negative significance to the placebo response and their desire always to rule it out blind them to its enormous positive potential and encourage them to propagate misconceptions about its nature. I regularly come across five major misconceptions about placebo responses when I talk about them with regular doctors and read the scientific medical literature.

Most medical doctors think that

1. placebo responses are not as strong as "objective" effects of treatments and can be differentiated from objective effects on that basis;
2. placebo responses are limited to certain kinds of people, usually called "placebo reactors" and characterized by certain psychological traits or educational or ethnic backgrounds;
3. only one kind of placebo exists — the sugar pill or its equivalent — that is, an inactive substance or a procedure with no significant intrinsic effects;
4. the efficacy of placebo treatments depends primarily on the belief of patients in them;
5. placebo responses can (and should) be ruled out by procedures such as double-blind drug testing, permitting clean separation of direct effects of treatments and indirect effects due to belief.

As far as the strength of the placebo response goes, it can be of any magnitude. There are placebo deaths and placebo cures of cancer. One kind of placebo death is known as voodoo death and has been the subject of psychiatric inquiry and even some physiological study by scientists willing to admit the power of the mind. Voodoo death occurs in some shamanistic societies, where, for one reason or another, malevolent witch doctors occasionally curse people. A person so cursed usually takes to his bed, stops eating, assumes a fatalistic attitude about his impending doom, withdraws from communication with family and friends, and dies, often within a week or two of learning of the curse.[5] Research on this phenomenon suggests a possible mechanism: abnormal overactivity of the parasympathetic nervous system, that branch of the autonomic or "involuntary" nervous system that slows down vital functions such as heartbeat and circulation. Evidently, the belief of a victim of voodoo death in the power of a witch doctor can find physical expression through the parasympathetic nerves, possibly resulting in eventual stoppage of the heart.[6]

There is no direct physical response of the human body to any therapeutic procedure that cannot occur with equal form and magnitude in response to an inert placebo. Placebos can relieve severe postoperative pain, induce sleep or mental alertness, bring about dramatic remissions in both symptoms and objective signs of chronic disease, initiate the rejection of warts and other abnormal growths, and so forth. They can equally elicit all the undesired consequences of treatment with real drugs, including nausea, headaches, skin rashes, hives and more serious allergic reactions, damage to organs, and addiction. (In this case they are sometimes called "nocebos," since their "effects" are noxious rather than pleasing.)[7]

It is incorrect to think that placebo responses are milder than direct effects of drugs or other treatments or to imagine that placebo responses can be distinguished from so-called objective responses by any consistent differences of form.

The second misconception of medical doctors, the existence of some subpopulation of placebo reactors distinct from the general population, is pure fantasy. Any person will respond to a placebo given under conditions that galvanize that individual's belief. It may be that the conventional dispensing of placebos by allopathic doctors who assign them negative significance does not inspire certain patients in the necessary way, but that does not mean those patients will not have placebo responses to other sorts of treatments coming from other sorts of practitioners.

Doctors have tried to construct a picture of the mythical placebo reactor. He or she is likely, they say, to be relatively uneducated, of neurotic disposition ("anxious, self-centered, and emotionally labile," in the words of one medical expert),[8] a regular churchgoer, of southern as opposed to northern European origin. On the other hand, "the trait that chiefly distinguishes those who seldom respond to the placebo is emotional stability. That and sophistication."[9]

This is utter nonsense. All serious research efforts to correlate particular personality traits with placebo responding have been unsuccessful.[10] Nor do I have any doubt where the amusing image comes from of an ignorant, hotheaded, neurotic, churchgoing Sicilian, who is supposed to be the archetypal placebo reactor. It comes from a desire to put as much distance as possible between the medical scientist proposing the concept and the kind of dupe who would fall for a sugar pill. As long as doctors think of placebo treatment as trickery, as a form of deception akin to quackery, they will not want to believe themselves capable of responding to it. Therefore, the placebo-resistant person will be emotionally stable, sophisticated, well-educated, altruistic, reserved, and preferably of Anglo-Saxon descent — just like the "perfect" physician.

As an example of a common placebo treatment that often works quite well in very sophisticated patients, including medical doctors, I might mention the prescription of antibiotics for sore throats of viral origin. The vast majority of ordinary sore throats are associated with viruses, not with bacteria, but antibiotics work against bacteria, having no power over viruses. Unless a throat culture demonstrates a specific bacterial infection in a case of sore throat, however severe or persistent, antibiotic therapy is not indicated. Yet it remains a very popular form of allopathic treatment, even when throat cultures are negative or when doctors do not bother to take them.

The use of antibiotics in this way is deplorable. It costs money, carries some medical risks, and worst of all, decreases the future effectiveness of the antibiotics by selecting resistant bacteria that may go out into the world and act as agents of disease in other people. Nevertheless, while condemning such treatment, I must admit that it sometimes works. I have collected many histories of patients with viral sore throats who experienced rapid cures within twenty-four to forty-eight hours of starting antibiotic therapy. In some cases the infections had persisted for days or weeks and refused to respond to other measures.

How does an antibiotic cure a viral sore throat? It can do so only by eliciting a placebo response, and the prevalence of such cures indicates the extent of real faith in the power of antibiotics on the part of both doctors and patients. Most of the patients in these histories were professional people, far from the stereotype of the placebo reactor. Some of them were physicians, who quickly got over their sore throats following self-medication with these drugs.

Of course, in this example, the remedies are hardly inert. Antibiotics are real drugs with intrinsic effects; however, those effects are irrelevant to the course of a viral infection. When an antibiotic cures a viral sore throat, it functions as a placebo apart from its own pharmacological activity. It is then an example of the "active placebo," to be explained in a moment. Of course, the activity and known power of these drugs are just what enable them to focus the belief of patients, including physicians and other highly educated people. Physicians may have little or no faith in sugar pills, homeopathic remedies, and acupuncture needles, but they are true believers in the power of antibiotics.

The third misconception of medical doctors concerns kinds of placebos. Most doctors do not consider active placebos and the great role they play in all forms of medical practice. They think of placebos only in the strict sense of inactive pills and procedures.

At first glance, "active placebo" might seem to be a contradiction, but it is an extremely useful concept, one that I will refer to frequently in these pages. The term is not of my invention, although I have worked to make it more popular. It was first used in connection with certain drug experiments where inactive placebos seemed inappropriate as controls.

One such investigation was a colorful piece of research called the Good Friday Experiment, held in the chapel of the Massachusetts Institute of Technology on Good Friday, 1962.[11] Its purpose was to determine whether a psychedelic drug, specifically psilocybin from magic mushrooms, could evoke genuine mystical experiences in human volunteers. The man who designed the experiment, Dr. Walter Pahnke, was a student of theology at Harvard University as well as an M.D. interested in the boundary between pharmacology and religion. His volunteers were other theology students, eager to have mystical experiences, who understood they would receive pills that might contain a drug associated with shamanistic ceremonies in Mexico. The experiences of people who eat the sacred mushrooms in these ceremonies have much in common with non-drug-related experiences of mystics in many other cultures. Dr. Pahnke arranged his experimental setting to favor such results, choosing the day and place accordingly, and heightening the expectations of his subjects with moving, religious music.

In order to find out whether psilocybin had any special ability to induce religious feelings, Pahnke wanted to use the double-blind method, giving half the volunteers psilocybin and half placebos, without his or their prior knowledge of which pills contained the mushroom drug. He foresaw a problem, however. Psilocybin is a very active pharmacological agent, producing easily perceptible psychosomatic changes. Like LSD (lysergic acid diethylamide) and other psychedelics, it is a strong stimulant of the central and sympathetic nervous systems. As a result, it directly causes wakefulness and distinctive bodily feelings, such as butterflies in the stomach, cold extremities, and a general sense of nervous excitement. Its effects on perception and mood are much less constant, but these symptoms of stimulation appear in most people who take the drug, and are of rapid onset and of such intensity that they rarely go unnoticed. Pahnke was not out to verify the intrinsic pharmacological activity of psilocybin but to test in a controlled fashion its capacity to evoke a particular experience. If some subjects were to feel strong drug effects within thirty minutes of the start of the experiment, while others felt nothing, it would soon be obvious to all who got the psilocybin, and that would spoil the test.

Pahnke dealt with this problem by using niacin as his placebo. Niacin (also called nicotinic acid) is a B-vitamin not known to have direct effects on the mind. No one has ever accused it of causing mystical experiences, but a large dose of it taken by mouth does cause a spectacular physical reaction. Within a half-hour or less it dilates small arteries near the surface of the body, bringing a great deal of blood to the skin. The first subjective awareness of this change is usually a feeling of warmth and prickling about the head and neck. It soon develops into a wave of intense flushing and stinging heat that spreads down the whole body and lasts from ten minutes to nearly an hour, turning into strong itching before it disappears. This reaction is quite harmless but dramatically intrudes itself on one's awareness while it runs its course.

Participants in the Good Friday Experiment all felt effects of the pills they took at about the same time. None of those who swallowed niacin had mystical experiences, although they believed they had taken some sort of drug. A significant percentage of those who received the psilocybin did have profound responses that Dr. Pahnke felt deserved to be called mystical and genuinely religious. He concluded that psilocybin could, indeed, produce such experiences by virtue of its special properties.

It is possible to criticize this experiment and Pahnke's conclusion. In fact, chapter 20 analyzes the relationship between psychoactive drugs and the experiences of people who take them in an effort to convince the reader that simple pharmacological cause and effect does not apply. Here I just wish to call attention to niacin as a classic example of an active placebo. Its intrinsic effects are dramatic, but since they are also irrelevant to the effect under study (mystical experience), niacin can be used legitimately as a standard of comparison for psilocybin in this double-blind experiment.

A moment's thought will help you realize that active placebos are much more common and much more important than inactive placebos. They are common because most medical treatments, both orthodox and unorthodox, have direct, perceptible effects and so convince patients something is happening to them. This belief, independent of all else, can initiate the placebo response. They are important because their activity makes them more convincing than pills that do nothing. Insertion of an acupuncture needle causes pain and other strong sensation. By that alone it may elicit a favorable placebo response independent of or in combination with any direct, beneficial effect it may have on illness. Similarly, an allopathic injection can easily function as an active placebo because the patient feels it and so is likely to believe in its power.

I am convinced that injections often elicit placebo responses by effectively getting attention and arousing strong emotions. Many people dislike or fear injections and try to avoid them. Many others love them and seek them out. Only persons who have no feelings about them — and I meet few of those — are unlikely to respond to them as active placebos. Whether attracted or repelled by needles, most people believe in their power, and that is all it takes to link them to the placebo response.

In traveling through rural areas of Mexico and Ecuador, I have often come across magical beliefs about injections. To primitive people, drugs injected by needle seem as wonderful and powerful as guns and distilled alcohol, the other symbols that make modern Western civilization look superior to traditional cultures. I have met villagers who made their livings as injectors, advertising their profession with crude drawings of syringes hung outside their huts. For a small fee, you could get an injection from one of these practitioners; what was in it was unimportant. I soon learned that the people who sought these treatments did not have much faith in their traditional herbal remedies or even in pharmaceutical pills. They wanted injections because they believed in their therapeutic magic. Often, they took drugs by injection that work perfectly well by mouth.

A friend in rural Nigeria sent me a description of a more remarkable version of the same belief. He watched itinerant injectors go from village to village, offering shots of colored water for a fee. Three colors were available — red, yellow, and blue — at different prices. Everyone knew the syringes contained nothing but colored water, and everyone who could afford it lined up to be injected when these curious practitioners came around.

When syringes contain active drugs that make people feel different, injections can be especially good at producing placebo responses, not just in remote villages but in modern hospitals, too. Let me recount another story, this one from a nurse who listened to me lecture about the placebo response. She had worked on a surgery ward in the days before disposable needles and syringes. In those days, glass syringes had to be sterilized by boiling and steel needles had to be sharpened for repetitive use. One of her patients was a difficult, middle-aged woman recovering from gall bladder removal. The surgeon had left a standing order for a nightly injection of pentobarbital (Nembutal) in case of insomnia. Since the woman could never sleep, the nurse found herself giving the injection regularly, but the patient's response to it was poor. She usually remained wakeful and complaining through much of the night.

One evening, the woman yelled and jumped on getting the shot. The nurse examined the needle afterward and noted that it was quite dull. Apparently, she had neglected to sharpen it. For the first time, the patient slept soundly. The nurse was alert enough to wonder whether these two observations might be connected. Over the next week, she gave the Nembutal injection with sharp and dull needles on alternate nights and proved to her own satisfaction that the efficacy of the treatment depended on whether it hurt or not. It was always the same dose of the same drug. Success or failure was determined by a factor other than the intrinsic pharmacological activity of the substance in the syringe. Doctors do not question the sedating effect of intramuscular Nembutal, and patients certainly perceive that effect. Still, an injection of a real drug can also function as an active placebo, with the needle contributing therapeutic power to the fluid flowing through it.

The fourth misconception of physicians is that the efficacy of placebo treatments depends primarily on the belief of patients.

In acknowledging the ability of antibiotics to produce occasional cures of viral sore throats, I called physicians true believers in the power of those drugs. The belief of doctors in the value of treatments is at least as important as the belief of patients.

When doctors prescribe inactive placebos, their knowledge of the inert nature of the pills leads them to interpret any therapeutic success as proof of the "power of suggestion" and the manipulability of patients' beliefs. This interpretation is also the source of the attitude that placebo treatment is deceptive and suspect in some way. In the narrow view of placebo responses to dummy pills, credulous patients are taken in by all-knowing doctors; the stereotype of the "placebo reactor" originates here.

Since patients will not feel any direct effects of sugar pills, their belief in the power of those pills must find other support. Research has shown inactive placebos to work better when they taste bitter or are very expensive, probably because bitter, expensive pills fit patients' preconceptions of drugs and so are more convincing. If a patient senses that a doctor believes a drug to be effective, that will also increase the chance of its working.

Oddly enough, doctors can tell some patients in so many words that the pills they are going to take contain nothing but sugar, and satisfactory placebo responses will still occur. This finding suggests that what a doctor tells a patient is less important than what the doctor feels and expresses nonverbally. The doctor who has seen the reality of placebo responses *knows* that sugar pills can produce every medical reaction from allergic shock to dramatic remission of chronic disease. That belief, communicated in some way, may overshadow an oral disclosure of inactivity. Beliefs of practitioners about treatments are crucial determinants of therapeutic outcomes.

The preceding remarks apply to the use of inactive placebos, when doctors know the pills are not real but patients usually do not. Think how much more effectively doctors will communicate their belief in the value of treatments when they really do believe in them. For that reason I maintain that active placebos can be much more powerful than inactive ones and can affect far more people. In addition to everything that goes on when a sugar pill is dispensed, the active placebo directly affects the patient, often in an immediately perceptible fashion (such as the sting of an injection), and carries the enormous influence of the doctor's own belief in it (antibiotics knock out infections; Nembutal puts people to sleep).

Regardless of the direct effects of therapeutic interventions, all of them can also function as active placebos, forcing the conclusion that any favorable outcome of any medical treatment may be due, at least in part, to a placebo response.

I am afraid this conclusion badly muddies the scientific evaluation of treatment. There is no practical way to eliminate all the elements of belief entering into therapy. Even the most careful double-blind experiments can only establish the efficacy of a new drug relative to an inactive control. Experiments cannot enable researchers to conclude how much of any specific instance of clinical success with that drug is due to direct pharmacological action and how much to a placebo response evoked indirectly by the combination of pharmacological action and belief in it. In fact, the success of a new drug in double-blind trials, by convincing doctors of intrinsic efficacy, will give it a thicker coating of belief and so increase its potential to elicit placebo responses.

I suppose doctors could let machines select and administer remedies to unconscious patients as a means of minimizing the role of belief, but even that might not do it. There would still be belief in the power of the machines, even at the unconscious level, and as I will show, it is the unconscious mind that controls the placebo response. Belief is of no consequence at the verbal, intellectual level unless it also penetrates the deeper strata of mind, often below conscious awareness, which connect to the physical nerves. Besides, what would be the point? Only a misguided passion for ruling out placebo phenomena could lead to such behavior. Not only is it theoretically impossible to do so, it is practically foolish, because as pure healing responses to therapeutic interventions, placebo reactions are the real meat of medicine. Doctors should worry about ruling them *in* rather than *out* and try to produce them more often by safe and effective means.

The negative significance assigned to placebo responses by conventional doctors leads them to regard these events as pesky problems to be eliminated. All of my understanding and experience lead me to the conclusion that the direct and indirect effects of treatments are inseparable. When a patient is treated and improvement results, no amount of thought, study, or experiment will permit doctors to draw sharp lines dividing mind-mediated responses from "objective" effects on the body. The root reason is the nonexistence of any such division between mind and body in the first place. Only if you imagine the mind to be unreal or unconnected to the body can you dream of ruling out placebo "effects." The fact of wart cures and other clear-cut examples of mind-mediated healing demonstrates the complete interpenetration of mind and body in ways yet to be described by science and of tremendous importance to the practice of medicine.

The fifth misconception among medical doctors about placebos is the most unproductive of all. Many doctors simply have not yet realized the positive significance of placebo responses: that they represent pure healing from within, free of the side effects and adverse reactions much more likely to be directly, causally related to treatment. I am all for controlled studies of drugs and other treatments to clarify their intrinsic actions. That information minimizes the chance of bringing dangerously active placebos (such as internal mammary artery ligation) into medical circulation. I have no interest, however, in trying to eliminate the placebo response in myself or in people who come to me as patients. The best treatments are those with safe and valuable intrinsic effects that focus the belief of both doctor and patient and so function well as active placebos, unblocking innate healing by a mind-mediated mechanism while also working directly on the body. This is psychosomatic medicine at its best and good medicine by any standard of judgment, not quackery or deception. In fact, the true art of medicine is the ability of a practitioner to select and present to individual patients those treatments most likely to elicit healing from within.*

---

*A few enlightened doctors have come to this realization and are attempting to convince their colleagues of it.[12]

20

Medical Treatments as Active Placebos

ONE OF THE FEW totally gratifying experiences I had as a medical intern was reviving a diabetic in insulin shock. He was a young man, brought unconscious by a friend to the emergency room of the San Francisco hospital where I worked. The friend had been with him when he injected himself with insulin a short time before. Apparently, the man had mistakenly given himself an overdose or failed to consider that he had not eaten enough beforehand. He had rapidly become weak and delirious, then lost consciousness.

The treatment for this medical emergency is specific. I filled a large syringe with a 50 percent solution of glucose, put the needle into a vein in the man's arm, and slowly injected sugar into his bloodstream. Within seconds he opened his eyes, moved, and regained normal consciousness enough to ask where he was and what had happened. Within minutes he was well enough to sit up and drink a glass of orange juice. Shortly afterward he went home. I have seldom been able to produce such immediate, spectacular cures of serious medical problems.

Here is a case where the placebo response seems irrelevant. The man was unconscious, his nervous system unable to function normally because an overdose of insulin had lowered his blood sugar below the needs of his brain cells. I gave specific treatment for the problem and feel confident in assuming that the increase in blood sugar caused his cure. I cannot say that mind-mediated healing had no role in this sequence of events, but I am willing to say it was minimal.*

*Of course, this medical emergency was an artificial condition brought about by unnatural administration of a powerful hormone. Most illness is not that simple in origin or that easy to reverse by specific therapy.

At the opposite extreme are successful absent healings by Christian Science practitioners. In those cases, no direct physical interventions take place, and recovery is entirely due to the placebo response.

Between these two extremes lie most interactions of patients and doctors. Practitioners apply methods they believe in — drugs, surgery, needles, manipulation, baths, herbs, diets, and so forth. The methods directly cause changes in the bodies of patients. Sometimes the changes are prominent and exert beneficial effects explainable in terms of known physical mechanisms (drugs and surgery). Sometimes the changes are obvious but any beneficial effects are unexplainable (bony manipulation). Sometimes successful treatments are not only unexplainable but do not even cause obvious changes (homeopathic remedies, acupuncture). In any case, all treatments can elicit placebo responses dependent on the beliefs of both practitioners and patients. Any direct beneficial effect of treatment can therefore be enhanced by an additional indirect effect — a halo of placebo response, if you will. There is no boundary between the two, and in most cases of successful treatment between the extremes of Christian Science practice and allopathic revival of a diabetic in insulin shock, no way even to decide which makes the greater contribution to the outcome.

My own favorable response to a homeopathic remedy falls into that broad category. I began this book by describing a personal experience with episodic pain in the upper gastrointestinal tract, presumptively diagnosed by a gastroenterologist as esophageal spasm and apparently cured by a homeopath who gave me a single dose of a very dilute preparation of sulfur, so dilute that it probably contained no sulfur. I feel comfortable with the conclusion that the homeopathic remedy functioned as an active placebo for me.

I am not willing to call it an inactive placebo, because the arguments of homeopaths for biological effects of their high-potency remedies are serious enough to warrant study by impartial investigators. Until I see better evidence for or against those effects, I cannot say what that dose of homeopathic sulfur might have done to me directly. Nor can I say what it might have done indirectly. I am the last person to be able to analyze my own deep beliefs and expectations of treatments, and for this situation, no one else can analyze them either. I am left with the answer that my cure was a response to an active placebo and am aware of all the uncertainty in those words. Most medical histories are no less free of uncertainty.

"One should use a new remedy as much as possible while it still has the power to heal." That perceptive recommendation is attributed to at least half a dozen different physicians of the nineteenth and early twentieth centuries, including Sir William Osler (1849–1919) of Johns Hopkins University. Its popularity and frequent quotation in medical writing indicate its aptness. In fact, new drugs most often produce favorable responses near the time of their introduction, when enthusiasm for them is highest. As time goes by, many of them work less and less well. Ten or twenty years later, physicians agree that they are not worth much and back away from their use. What changes? Not the drugs or their pharmacology. The only possible answer lies in declining belief in their value on the part of physicians (and manufacturers) and, secondarily, of patients. As belief in a new drug fades, so does its potential to serve as an active placebo. The bright halo surrounding its direct actions evaporates, leaving them standing alone and suddenly looking not very impressive.*

Studies of psychoactive drugs reveal them to be model active placebos, since all of the interesting experiences users report

*A recent example of this process is declining effectiveness of the painkiller propoxyphene (Darvon), widely prescribed by medical doctors when it was first introduced in 1957. Although the drug was a synthetic opiate, its manufacturer promoted it as nonaddicting and nonnarcotic, and doctors welcomed it as a safe and useful analgesic, intermediate in strength between aspirin and morphine. Combinations of propoxyphene with aspirin and other standard analgesics also became available; these combinations achieved greater popularity than plain Darvon. By the 1970s, enthusiasm for this drug began to wane. Its abuse potential became obvious when heroin addicts who liked to inject it intravenously were discovered. Then, both patients and doctors started to question whether Darvon really relieved pain as well as older drugs. Many doctors now feel that Darvon combinations work mostly because they contain aspirin or acetaminophen. As belief in the value of propoxyphene eroded, so did its ability to work as a painkiller in terms of the percentage of patients reporting satisfactory effects from it. Doctors tend not to see the diminishing placebo returns as a change but rather to think the drug was not very good from the start and longer experience has made its limitations clear.

from them, whether positive or negative, seem to be products more of expectation and setting than of pharmacology. People who take psilocybin and LSD sometimes have mystical experiences, but some people also have mystical experiences when they pray, meditate, fast, or suffer severe illness. The experiences of many people who take these drugs are quite devoid of mystical or religious feelings. Therefore, mystical experience looks like a capacity of the human mind rather than the effect of any drug.

A theology student who longs to meet God face to face, who believes that an exotic Mexican mushroom might provide the means, and who takes psilocybin in a chapel on Good Friday with the music of Wagner's *Parsifal* swelling in the background might well have his longing fulfilled. It is fair to conclude that psilocybin can evoke religious experiences *under certain conditions of set (expectation) and setting*, but I consider it a waste of time to look for an underlying pharmacological mechanism. That niacin is ineffective in the same circumstances means that the intrinsic activity of that vitamin is less consistent with mystical experience than the intrinsic activity of psilocybin. Remember that psilocybin is quite active: the stimulation and perceptual changes it causes by its direct actions on the nervous system are consistent with euphoria and radical shifts in consciousness. The flushing caused by niacin is much less so.

Experiences of people who take psychoactive drugs with sedative effects (such as alcohol, barbiturates, and tranquilizers) are likely to be different from those of people who take psychedelics because they will be shaped by sedation rather than stimulation of the central nervous system. The experiences of people who smoke marijuana are astounding in their variety because marijuana has such slight intrinsic activity compared to other substances and is neither a pronounced sedative nor a stimulant. Some users can smoke pot as an aid to sleep, while others take it to concentrate on tasks. Some become hilariously extroverted on it, others morosely introverted. Some find it decreases interest in sex; others consider it an aphrodisiac. Some use it for meditation; others become mentally scattered under its influence. There is no unifying theme to these reactions except that they are largely conditioned by set and setting rather than by the unimpressive pharmacology of marijuana.

In general, the stronger a psychoactive drug and the more specific its activity, the greater will be the role of pharmacology in shaping responses to it. Even with very strong drugs, however, set and setting remain crucial variables.

I once reviewed cases of intoxication by a wild mushroom called the panther amanita (*Amanita pantherina*), which grows abundantly in the woods of western Oregon and Washington. Mushroom books call it seriously poisonous and include stern warnings of its dangers. Occasionally, mushroom hunters eat it inadvertently, mistaking it for an edible species. In recent years, other people have eaten it deliberately, hoping to get high by doing so.*

The panther amanita contains two very active drugs, ibotenic acid and muscimol, that rapidly affect the nervous system. These compounds are sedating, producing easily perceptible changes in body feelings, muscle coordination, and mental state. In high doses the direct effects are quite unpleasant, often culminating in a delirium that can lead to accidental injury, but they are not life-threatening and subside within twenty-four hours as the body metabolizes and eliminates the responsible chemicals. In moderate doses ibotenic acid and muscimol cause definite intoxication, but how people experience it is clearly determined by set and setting.

Foragers who cook up a meal of these mushrooms by mistake usually realize their error quickly, decide they are poisoned, and think they are about to die. They experience physical sickness, fear, disorientation, and, often, temporary loss of consciousness. If they go to emergency rooms of hospitals, they are likely to

*They were inspired by reports of the psychoactivity of a close relative, the fly agaric, *Amanita muscaria*. This striking red mushroom with white dots on its cap contains unusual chemical compounds and has been suggested in popular books as the botanical identity of *soma*, an intoxicant used ceremonially by ancient Aryan peoples of India. The panther amanita looks similar but is brown instead of red. In the early 1970s, after scientists reported it contained higher doses of the same chemicals, the first cases of deliberate ingestion of the panther amanita by persons seeking psychoactive effects came to the attention of mushroom experts.

receive heroic treatments that make them feel worse and confirm their fears of medical disaster.*

Those who eat the same mushroom deliberately rarely become sick, do not seek treatment or help, often enjoy their experiences, and occasionally repeat them. They describe pleasant, dreamlike states, unusual perceptions, and various forms of "heightened consciousness."

Unquestionably, this curious fungus works as an active placebo, its direct effects serving to elicit both positive and negative experiences. Many mushroom hunters are profoundly and unconsciously afraid of being poisoned. Those who eat the panther amanita by mistake and soon feel the direct actions of ibotenic acid and muscimol can easily turn them into the symptoms of fatal mushroom poisoning, concentrating on their disruptive aspects and thereby intensifying them. Such people create sickness from the intoxication, becoming terrified themselves and acting in ways that make others terrified about their condition.

Seekers of new natural highs interpret the same direct actions of the same drugs very differently. They welcome them as signs that "something is happening," concentrate on what they perceive as the pleasant aspects, use them as opportunities for altered states of consciousness, and ignore or forget any unpleasant effects.

Even the problems people have with narcotics are strongly influenced by expectation and setting. Pharmacologists give us the idea that drug craving and addiction are unvarying consequences of repetitive use of opiates, but medical patients who become accidentally addicted in the course of hospitalization do not experience the kind of euphoria from narcotics that nonmedical users do, nor do they have great trouble with withdrawal and abstinence. On the other hand, some street addicts,

---

*Until very recently, handbooks of emergency medicine recommended treating panther amanita intoxication with large injections of atropine. Atropine is a drug from nightshade-family plants that antagonizes the effects of muscarine, erroneously believed to be the active principle of this mushroom. In fact, the panther amanita contains little if any muscarine, and atropine potentiates the actions of the drugs it does contain. Unlucky patients who got shots of atropine in emergency rooms as treatment for poisoning by this mushroom experienced immediate intensification of all their symptoms, while the doctors who ordered the shots probably saw in these reactions further cause for alarm and need to intervene.

when they cannot obtain drugs, inject themselves with water and get satisfying effects from the injections.

During the Vietnam War, a very high percentage of American soldiers in Southeast Asia used heroin every day, smoking it as a means of escaping the boredom of military life. In the special setting of Vietnam, a combination of extreme boredom and easy availability of cheap, strong heroin seduced many men into habitual use of narcotics. Pharmacology predicted that most of those men would have to keep on using opiates when they returned home, swelling the ranks of domestic addicts. In fact, that did not happen. Even after months of heavy use, most soldiers simply ended their involvement with opiates when they came back to the United States and different conditions. Withdrawal and recidivism were not problems for them.[1]

I have also collected some interesting cases of placebo withdrawal in patients at methadone maintenance clinics. For example, a thirty-two-year-old male heroin addict, who entered methadone maintenance with high motivation to end his career as an addict, was told his dose of oral methadone would be progressively cut to zero over a three-month period. Each day he was to take a pill, but the pills would have less and less of the narcotic and eventually would contain none at all. He expressed fear of withdrawal and doubts of his ability to handle reality without opiates but agreed to try this graduated reduction of dose as long as he did not know exactly when he would have to begin to face life unaided. At the end of six weeks, his daily pill became a completely inert placebo. He showed no withdrawal symptoms at that time. After another four weeks, a staff doctor told him he had been off methadone totally for a month. On receiving the news, the man suddenly went into withdrawal, showing classic symptoms — muscle cramps, gooseflesh, a runny nose, and general mental and physical discomfort.

Psychoactive drugs are model active placebos because they really do make people feel different, and because the feelings they give are neutral and ambivalent, lending themselves to the creative interpretation and shaping of individual users. It is activity perceptible to both patient and doctor that enables drugs to work as better placebos than sugar pills. Therefore, more active drugs will also be more likely to work indirectly through the mind. A drug that produces nausea or dizziness, or an injection that leaves the arm sore, is a convincing treatment. So is any form of surgery. If a mere injection can elicit a placebo response, the mind-focusing power of a full-scale operation, with all of its drama and violation of the body, must be formidable. Any surgery, in addition to its direct effect, is likely to generate a placebo response.

Strong treatments such as surgery make good active placebos, both because they impress patients and because allopathic doctors have greatest faith in techniques with high impact on the physical body. Unfortunately, strong treatments are also more likely to cause harm. If the placebo response can be more important in determining a medical outcome than the direct effect of a drug or procedure, then any direct injury is especially unjustifiable. In other words, the trauma of surgery is hard to defend if nonsurgical treatment will give an equally favorable placebo response.

Finding a suitable balance between treatments strong enough to convince patients of efficacy but not do them serious harm is hard. It depends on the prevailing beliefs in any society about the nature of illness and treatment.

In our society, widespread faith in technology and the importance of physical reality makes relatively traumatic procedures more effective at mobilizing mind-mediated healing than relatively gentle ones. This fact is sad, but it is a fact. It explains why naturopathy is a weak competitor with allopathy today and why Bach flower remedies are not likely to work for the mass of Americans who go to regular doctors. Certainly, most regular doctors will never see such treatments as anything other than inactive placebos and so will be unable to communicate their belief in them to patients.

The contribution of doctors' beliefs to the therapeutic process cannot be overestimated. Their conviction of the value of what they do to patients is all-important. I recognize three dimensions of belief in placebo responses to active treatments: the patient's belief in the method, the doctor's belief in the method, and the patient's and doctor's belief in each other.* If all of these factors

*An almost identical statement is attributed to the Dalai Lama. In discussing the herbal remedies of traditional Tibetan medicine with a Harvard Medical School physician, he is quoted as saying that three elements are essential to their success: "the belief of the patient, the belief of the doctor, and the 'karma' between the two."[2]

work optimally, even procedures based on ridiculous theories can produce real cures. If they do not interact productively, even the most scientific and rational treatments may fail to cure.

An explanation for the conclusions stated in chapter 17 about the various medical systems examined earlier is that the additive beliefs of patients and practitioners in particular methods and in each other can produce curative placebo responses even if the methods arise from theories easily refuted by science. Thus any system of treatment, potentially, can produce real cures, even of organic disease.

Conversely, the failure of three-way belief to interact productively would explain some failures of treatments, even those based on scientifically valid principles. Inconsistency among systems of treatment is of no consequence, because the direct effects of any method may be dwarfed by placebo responses dependent on mutual belief. The early success and later decline of prominent medical heresies is the same process that occurs with new drugs: efficacy fades over time as belief of doctors and patients in them diminishes.

Some perceptive scholars believe the history of medicine is actually the history of the placebo response. I agree with them. Contemporary physicians are likely to dismiss the remedies of the distant past, such as powdered mummies and crabs' eyes, as "nothing more" than placebos, but they are less likely to concede that the drugs and procedures of modern allopathy also owe much or most of their value to placebo responses. Their resistance comes from failure to distinguish between inactive and active placebos and to see that the most active treatments will have the brightest placebo halos. Ironically, it is the faith of today's doctors in their powerful drugs and operations that helps provide those halos.

As medical beliefs change over time, placebo responses will also change, forming new associations with treatments. Just as doctors and patients can lose faith in a drug like Darvon, they can gain it in a procedure like acupuncture. At the moment, some important discoveries about brain chemistry are leading allopaths to change their beliefs about placebos, possibly signaling a new era of treatment in which placebos will have greater status. These discoveries are worth summarizing.

The cornerstone of modern neurochemical theory, dating back only to about 1950, is the principle that chemicals exert their actions on nerves by fitting into special receptor sites on nerve cells, just as keys fit into locks. For a chemical to carry some message to a nerve, its molecule must have a three-dimensional structure allowing it to occupy a specialized receptor designed to fit that molecule or one very much like it. The drug-receptor combination, once made, can affect the function of the cell, for example by increasing or decreasing its likelihood to fire an electrical impulse down its outgoing fiber. This theory is supported by much experimental evidence, including the precise localization of receptors for particular neurochemicals in particular areas of the brain.

Pharmacologists have known for some time that drugs such as morphine and codeine attach to special opiate receptors on some brain cells, and they have begun to identify the common three-dimensional configurations of natural and synthetic narcotics that suggest the complementary structure of the opiate receptor. They also now understand the mechanism of action of other drugs called narcotic antagonists that block the effects of opiates if given before them. One such drug, naloxone, will prevent morphine or heroin from having any effect and will also immediately precipitate withdrawal in an opiate addict. Evidently, narcotic antagonists are like keys that fit easily in locks but do not turn. They have a high affinity to bind to opiate receptors, but they do not affect the activity of the nerve cells on their own and, once in place, prevent molecules of narcotics from attaching to the same sites.

These facts raise an interesting question. Why should the brain have receptors for opiate molecules in the first place? Medical scientists often refuse to consider such questions, dismissing them as teleological. That is, they have to do with the final purposes of the design of the universe and supposedly, therefore, lie beyond the reasonable concerns of science. Some researchers *have* troubled themselves wondering why the human brain has receptors designed to fit molecules made by poppy plants. They proposed an interesting hypothesis: perhaps opiate receptors in the brain are really there to interact with molecules made by the brain itself, molecules that just happen to resemble those in opium.

Investigation of this possibility led in 1975 to the discovery of a family of substances called endorphins. *Endorphin* is a coined word meaning "the morphine within." These substances are chemically distinct from poppy drugs but share with them some three-dimensional structure that allows them to bind with opiate receptors. They exert typical opiatelike effects. Pharmacologists also call them endogenous opioids, meaning "opiatelike substances made within [the body]."

This discovery is a momentous step in understanding neurochemical mechanisms. Endorphins are now the subject of intensive research that may have many practical applications. For example, it may clarify the problems of opiate addiction and suggest new treatments for it. Perhaps people who like opiates and are drawn to using them addictively have a deficiency of endorphins, causing them to perceive ordinary irritations as too painful to bear. Perhaps the regular use of external opiates shuts off the production of the endogenous painkillers. In that case, the withdrawal syndrome would be a manifestation of a sudden, drastic lack of opiates or opioids, which might play some vital role in the economy of the central nervous system. Perhaps ways can be found to stimulate internal production of endorphins as a better approach to treating addiction.

Another possibility is that endorphins mediate some psychosomatic events that have baffled medical scientists up to now. The ability of some people to tolerate pain that most people cannot may represent an efficient endorphin system. Since inactive placebos are mostly used to relieve pain and since they do so quite effectively in a sizable fraction of patients, it is tempting to think they somehow cause the release of endorphins. Maybe endorphins also explain the mystery of acupuncture anesthesia.

The involvement of endorphins in analgesia and anesthesia produced by placebos and acupuncture has now been confirmed by experimental demonstrations of the power of narcotic antagonists to block the effects. Naloxone interferes substantially with the pain-relieving properties of both sugar pills and Chinese needles.[3] A logical conclusion is that endorphins mediate any satisfactory responses to these treatments.

This finding has enormous theoretical and practical significance. It suddenly takes certain placebo responses — relief of pain by inert pills — out of the realm of the mystical and makes them fully accessible to doctors and researchers who need physical handles. Identification of a biochemical mechanism for placebo analgesia has done more to change the image of placebos than any amount of arguing about the importance of belief and the mind. The mind may still seem unreal to many allopaths, but it can suppress pain by activating a mechanism involving real molecules.

There is now a tendency to invoke endorphins as explanations for all sorts of other mysterious phenomena, from fire walking to faith healing. I am sure the full story of the brain's own narcotics is just beginning to emerge, but I am afraid many of these explanations are just wild guesses that will not hold up. Although opiates help cure a few diseases, notably colds, flus, and some intestinal problems, they do not produce anything resembling the range of placebo responses seen in clinical medicine. There is no reason to think endorphins are responsible for powers of placebos beyond the relief of pain or for healing in response to unorthodox treatments. Other mechanisms, yet to be discovered, may underlie more complex mind-body interactions. If one has come to light, I am optimistic that others will, gradually removing the appearance of unreality that has deterred scientists from taking these phenomena seriously.

I hope that research on endorphins will enable doctors to see the substance in placebo responses and appreciate their virtue. I hope, particularly, they will come to see placebo medicine not as trickery but as a valid means of activating mind-controlled mechanisms of internal healing. Then they might begin to use inactive placebos more creatively, prescribing them enthusiastically and with good intent, instead of ordering them ambivalently for disliked patients.

Even if these changes come about, I fear that understanding of the prevalence and power of active placebos will lag behind for several reasons. First, no practitioner wants to admit any intrinsic weakness of his or her methods. Just as homeopaths bristle at hearing their remedies put down as placebos, so will chiropractors resist the idea that bony manipulation of the spine is more likely to exert beneficial effects indirectly rather than directly, and so will allopaths insist that when their drugs work, direct pharmacological actions are responsible.

Second, the concept of the active placebo is peculiarly difficult for dualists because it denies any clean separation between mind and body. I repeat my contention that it is simply impossible ever to know where objective effects of treatments leave off and placebo responses begin. When the antibiotic tetracycline produces a rapid cure of a viral sore throat, I rate the placebo response uppermost but will not deny a role for the activity of the drug. It alters bacterial flora in the body, possibly changing tissue chemistry in the throat, possibly changing the state of the immune system, possibly providing subtle pharmacological cues to the patient that help mobilize internal healing. There is no hope of exactly defining its contribution to the cure.

On the other hand, when tetracycline produces a rapid cure of a lower urinary tract infection associated with susceptible bacteria, it is tempting to rate the direct antibiotic effect of treatment uppermost and ignore the placebo response. In many cases that estimation may be true, but again, there is no way to know. Tetracycline does not always cure infections it ought to. Perhaps when it succeeds, its direct actions give the body an advantage over the germs, an advantage on which the placebo response can capitalize in order to effect total cure by innate mechanisms of healing.

This logical difficulty leads some people to make light of active placebos. "Well, then, everything is a placebo," a reader might say. Yes, I suppose that is true or, at least, potentially true. It does not invalidate the concept. Others will protest that they *know* certain drugs and treatments are "real" (as if *real* were the opposite of *placebo*). Marijuana smokers often object vigorously to my calling their favorite drug an active placebo. "You just haven't tried any really good pot," some of them tell me. That comment is just like the protestation of the asthmatic who insists, "My asthma is real!" when someone calls it "psychosomatic." Of course, asthma is real, as are the changes that follow smoking marijuana. All of the evidence suggests, however, that the experiences pot smokers like are capacities of the mind, which become associated with the subtle psychophysical effects directly caused by the drug.

The association is not automatic. People must learn to get

high on marijuana. Until the association forms, they may notice
nothing at all from smoking it, even from smoking large doses.
That was exactly the experience of volunteer subjects to whom
I gave the drug in double-blind experiments in Boston in 1968.[4]
Never having had marijuana before and receiving no encouragement from set and setting, they simply felt nothing from it,
although their heart rates increased and the whites of their eyes
turned red, reflecting the drug's direct actions. At the other
extreme are people who smoke marijuana all the time and also
have no significant experiences from it. As a result of overuse,
the slight direct effects of the drug lose all novelty for them,
sink below perceptible levels, and no longer can serve to elicit
desired mental states — the placebo responses many users think
come from outside.

Marijuana, like all recreational drugs, is an active placebo that
works for those people who come to like it. More active drugs,
such as alcohol and heroin, may require less learning because
their stronger direct effects are more noticeable, but the relationship between their pharmacology and the psychological states
users seek from them is the same indirect one that allows people
to feel high (or paranoid or mystical or erotic or crazy) from
smoking pot.

I have written at length elsewhere about psychoactive drugs
and experiences associated with them.[5] Rather than repeat myself, I will just note that the concept of medical treatments as
active placebos is an expansion of the same idea. "Drug highs"
are really latent in the mind, waiting to be released by substances
that push people in certain psychopharmacological directions
but work as desired only if set and setting interact with pharmacology to produce the release. In the same way, healing is an
innate, latent capacity of the mind-body, waiting to be released
or unblocked by methods that may directly give sick people a
hand in overcoming illness but succeed only if the beliefs of both
patients and practitioners interact productively with them.

A third difficulty with the concept of the active placebo is our
great ignorance about the nature of mind and brain, the relationship between them, and the ways they influence the body.
Discovery of the endorphin system provides a glimpse of one
mechanism by which belief may cause dramatic alterations in

our experience of physical reality. Until we uncover other mechanisms of mind-body interactions, the subject of active placebos will continue to look hopelessly vague to many people and discouragingly mystical to most scientists. I stress mechanisms not because I am a mechanist but because I see them as keys to changes in attitudes about research on and use of the placebo response as the central element of healing and successful treatment.

Whatever may be the direct effect of a drug, surgical operation, or other physical intervention given by a medical practitioner to a sick person with the intention of promoting cure, it can also indirectly bring about healing by eliciting a placebo response. Placebo responses may result in total cure in combination with, independent of, or in spite of the direct effect of treatment. It is impossible ever to specify the individual contributions of these two aspects of therapy.

All practitioners of all systems of medicine should regard the placebo response as a therapeutic ally and work to evoke it more of the time, no matter what methods they use and how confident they are of their direct beneficial effects.

21

*Powers of the Mind and
the Problem of Harnessing Them*

THIS CHAPTER DESCRIBES a few examples of extraordinary mind-mediated phenomena I have studied or experienced personally. I do not understand them in terms of psychophysical mechanisms or know how to produce them on command, but I believe they represent capacities of all human beings and are not beyond scientific analysis. Eventually, their details will come to light. They should inspire doctors to find more ways of treating the ills of the body by taking advantage of powers of the mind and convince patients that those powers are always available to help restore lost health.

Psychosomatic Effects of Hypnosis

Hypnosis is real and important, despite its checkered past. Its relationship to medicine has always been uneasy, cycling through periods of cautious acceptance and indignant rejection. As a healing technique it has never shaken off the aura of charlatanism associated with its first modern exponent, Franz Anton Mesmer (1734–1815). Mesmer was an Austrian physician who recognized the power of suggestion to affect the physical body and tried to remove it from the mystical context of faith healing. In his view, faith healing made use of a perfectly natural energy, unrelated to any holiness of the healer or faith of the sufferer. He called this energy "animal magnetism," believing it to be related to physical magnetism, and he developed a curious healing ritual to make use of it. He had patients sit in a circle around a large tub of iron filings. Each patient held a rod projecting from the tub, while Mesmer and his assistants used hypnotic techniques to heighten suggestibility and expectations of healing. In this way, he was able to produce real cures of both functional and organic diseases.

Mesmer's manner alienated orthodox physicians, and his success and popularity outraged them. A scientific commission appointed by the French government to investigate his practice denounced him vigorously. It did not deny his cures but concluded they were the results of patients' imaginations rather than the workings of his tub. Therefore, it branded Mesmer a charlatan, completely missing the point that cures achieved by imagination have great medical significance, at least as much as cures produced by drugs and surgery.[1] Not until more than sixty years after Mesmer's death did the French Academy of Medicine recognize therapeutic uses of hypnosis. Not until 1958 did the American Medical Association officially declare hypnosis to have a secure place in modern medical practice.

Not only is hypnosis tainted by association with kooks, quacks, and stage artists, it is also hard to study, because it is essentially an altered state of consciousness, not an altered state of physiology, and so is unmeasurable by the methods of medical research. Therefore, it remains mystical and unreal for materialists and seems to them more appropriate as a theatrical entertainment than a technique of scientific medicine.

Many contradictory words about hypnosis are in print. It is a subject that inspires passionate debate as to what it is and how to use it. I am uninterested in most of these arguments but very interested in certain psychosomatic effects easily observable in good hypnotic subjects, effects that demonstrate the power of suggestion to modify bodily functions usually considered involuntary and beyond the reach of consciousness.

For instance, hypnosis can change the response of skin to thermal stimulation. It can increase or decrease the extent of redness and blistering resulting from contact with hot objects and can even cause skin to react with the usual signs of a burn to the touch of a cool object that the hypnotist suggests to be hot. These effects are mediated by nerves controlling small arteries in the skin. People cannot will changes in them, which makes their inclusion in the involuntary, or autonomic, nervous system seem logical. Yet hypnotic induction and suppression of burns demonstrate that circuits exist to convey suggestions from the mind to those nerves — sufficient proof that involuntary functions are potentially subject to mental influence.

Many other hypnotic demonstrations reinforce this conclusion and make it clear that neural links connect the entire autonomic nervous system to the higher brain and mind. How and under what circumstances those connections operate remain to be discovered, but they must contribute to the psychosomatic nature of all health and all disease and must also explain some of the power of belief to determine the outcome of treatment.

Voluntary Control of Internal States

Other sorts of evidence support that of hypnosis. Adepts at yoga are often able to demonstrate remarkable voluntary control of their digestive, respiratory, and circulatory systems. They say they acquire these abilities by practicing mental and physical exercises, particularly by regulating breath. Breathing is unique in being under the control of both voluntary and involuntary nerves. Possibly, yogic breathing exercises provide a bridge between these two systems, giving the will access to nerves and functions ordinarily closed to it.

In recent years, doctors interested in teaching patients to gain voluntary control of internal states have searched for techniques more reliable than hypnosis and requiring less work than yoga. Some of them have made use of forms of meditation that allow patients to relax the tone of autonomic nerves and thereby lower blood pressure and relieve stress on the heart, stomach, and intestines.[2] Others have worked with the simple, new method called biofeedback that lets patients monitor the functions they wish to control. In a common form of biofeedback training, people learn to increase blood flow to their hands by relaxing the autonomic nerves that regulate it. They pay attention to the skin temperature of their fingers, which is converted to an audio or visual display in order to provide continuous feedback. If temperature is indicated by the rate of a clicking sound, the trainee's job is to increase the rate of the clicks. Without having any idea what they are doing, people quickly get the knack of speeding up the clicks and, indirectly, of warming their fingers by allowing more blood to flow to them. With a little practice, they can then do it on their own, no longer needing the input from the biofeedback machine.[3]

The nerves that regulate superficial blood flow are part of the sympathetic nervous system, that branch of the autonomic nervous system that prepares the body for emergencies by conserving energy and directing it to vital functions. Constricting small arteries in the skin is part of this preparation because it makes more blood available for other organs. By learning to increase blood flow to their hands through biofeedback training, people are able to reap benefits greater than warm fingers. Increased sympathetic tone is the root of a number of chronic disorders of circulation and digestion, including high blood pressure, irregularities of heart rhythm, and spastic conditions of the stomach and colon. Doctors interested in psychosomatic medicine have long suspected that unexpressed (and even unconscious) feelings of anger and anxiety might cause the sympathetic nervous system to react as if a real emergency threatened from outside and so maintain the body in a chronic state of internal tension. Whatever the causes, abnormally high tone in these nerves subjects many organs to stress, resulting first in functional disease and eventually in organic changes.

Biofeedback provides a safe and effective means of dealing with these conditions. I like it also because it does not make patients dependent on outside help. In fact, it shows them how to manage their own bodies in new ways and so increases medical self-reliance. In some cases it acts as specific therapy for diseases not easily managed by standard allopathic techniques. Raynaud's disease is one of these. It is a condition of unknown origin, marked by unbalanced functioning of the sympathetic nerves controlling arterial blood flow to the extremities, especially the hands. Raynaud's disease mostly afflicts young women and expresses itself as attacks of painful blanching of the fingers on exposure to cold or during emotional upsets. In these episodes, blood flow to the fingers (and sometimes the toes) is severely reduced. The disease is progressive, can result in damage to the nails and skin, and sometimes travels with other, more serious, chronic diseases that affect structures throughout the body.*

*Systemic lupus erythematosus (SLE), for example.

Allopaths have used both drugs and surgery to try to relieve Raynaud's disease, often without much success or at the expense of causing more trouble than they cure. (The surgical approach is to cut major sympathetic nerve trunks, a procedure with many uncomfortable side effects.) I consider biofeedback training to be the treatment of choice for this condition.

Aside from their therapeutic applications, biofeedback and other methods of learning voluntary control of internal states force the conclusion that mind can influence body in far more ways than medical scientists have thought. Possibly, no physiological function is absolutely involuntary. Possibly, consciousness can reach every organ, tissue, and cell through the brain and nerves. Possibly, some physical limitations we now accept as immutable constraints on the human body are, in fact, plastic and subject to the power of the mind.

A "Miracle Cure" of Cancer

This history concerns a woman friend, whose cancer and cure ran their courses under the full scrutiny of allopathic physicians and surgeons in a university teaching hospital. I use it as an example because I know the patient and consider the case well documented.

When S.R., a twenty-six-year-old white female, noticed a painless lump in her neck in November 1967, she was extremely unhappy in her marriage and in her involvement with a doctoral program of experimental psychology concerned with animal behavior. She was also two months pregnant with her seventh pregnancy, all of the previous six having ended in miscarriages. Biopsy showed the lump to be an enlarged lymph node filled with malignant cells. A diagnosis of Hodgkin's disease, a cancer of the lymphatic system, was made. Out of a possible four stages of worsening prognosis, S.R.'s case was rated at "stage 3" because cancerous nodes were found both above and below the diaphragm — in the groin as well as in the neck and chest.

The patient's physician urged her to have an immediate abortion and a course of radiation therapy with X-rays. She refused, saying she desperately wanted the baby. He gave her the choice of following his orders or finding another doctor.

S.R. traveled to another city and found a physician at a university hospital who treated many cancer patients and was willing to let her continue the pregnancy. On his advice, she had surgery to remove the malignant nodes from her groin and a course of radiocobalt therapy directed at her chest, a treatment less likely to injure the fetus than X-rays. At this time, the patient's appetite disappeared, and her weight dropped sharply. She began to lose ground so fast that the doctor feared she might not live long enough to have the baby.

The doctor was not an average physician, being much concerned with the mind and its relationship to disease. He encouraged the patient to begin talking about her unhappiness, then tried to make her see she was acting out a desire to die. He also tried to get her interested in the problems of other people, inviting her to put her background in psychology to use by helping him interview patients, including those with advanced cancers.

Following the radiation treatment, S.R. lost all her hair and developed a stubborn respiratory infection. She had to be hospitalized and went into another phase of rapid decline. Her weight dropped to ninety-two pounds. As she lost her physical strength, her mental outlook also worsened. She remembers being apathetic about her condition, not caring if she lived or died.

It happened that her doctor was studying the use of the psychedelic drug LSD in terminal cancer patients, a procedure reported to help some of them adjust to the imminence of death when combined with supportive psychotherapy. He persuaded the patient to undergo a guided LSD trip in the hospital once her acute infection was under control, not for the purpose of reconciling her to death but to try to change her negative state of mind.

During this LSD experience, the doctor encouraged the patient to go inside herself and attempt to get in touch with the life of the baby in her womb. Under the influence of the drug and his guidance, she was able to do so. He then asked her if she had any right to cut off that life. S.R. recalls having a sudden and overwhelming realization that she had a choice as to whether she lived or died. She decided then and there she wanted to live and understood that she faced a struggle back to life that would require all her energy.

In the days and weeks following this flash of illumination, she made a number of major changes in her life. She left her husband, moved to her parents' home, dropped experimental psychology and enrolled in a program of clinical psychology, began working with a doctor famed for her studies of death and dying, and under her supervision worked with other patients with cancer. She took Gestalt psychology training with an encounter group, got a practitioner of Zen to advise her on meditation, and began to visualize energy flowing around her body. She also changed her diet radically, eliminating sugar and learning to eat mainly raw foods.

S.R. quickly rallied, gaining weight and strength. In June of 1968 she gave birth to a normal girl, then had a course of X-ray therapy. She says she does not know what did it — the radiation, diet, mental exercises, or life changes — but no new cancerous nodes appeared, and those that had been there disappeared.

That September, two new malignant nodes developed in her neck. These were removed surgically, and she had another course of X-rays. At this time she was on a strict raw-food diet and was practicing meditation and visualization every day.

In 1973 a questionable node appeared in her abdomen, but recurrence of cancer was not confirmed. Since then, S.R. has had no evidence of disease. She has remarried and had another healthy child. Physically, she is transformed. Her hair regrew curly and red; what fell out had been straight and black. She is now a vibrant, healthy woman, who works as a counselor of patients with advanced cancer. Her doctor says she is his best-documented miracle cure. She says she has no doubt that people with serious illness choose whether to live or die, even if they are unaware of making the choice.

There is no question in S.R.'s mind or mine that the healing process began with the flash of insight during the LSD trip, an event similar to a religious conversion. That motivated her to get well and look for ways to restore her health. Radiation, surgery, a raw-food diet, change of mate and career, meditation and visualization — all might have helped bring about the happy result of a cure. It is impossible to know what did what, but the change in consciousness was basic. Without that, her disease might have continued to progress no matter what measures were applied.

I should note that Hodgkin's disease, like some leukemias, may be more easily influenced than many other cancers. It has a higher tendency to remission, both spontaneous and induced, and may be more responsive to mental changes. I should also note that LSD has no intrinsic ability to initiate healing or to modify the course of any form of cancer. Under optimal conditions of set and setting it can favor flashes of meaningful insight, and in this case it worked splendidly. It might or might not work in others. There are reports of similar conversions and cures initiated by intense prayer, visits to miracle shrines, and contact with religious healers.

Whatever initiates it and however it works, a dramatic change in consciousness can affect the course of an illness for the better, even a very serious illness like Hodgkin's disease.

Some Noteworthy Experiences of People Who Take Psychedelic Drugs

As a result of my long interest in hallucinogenic plants and their derivatives, I have had occasion to take LSD and related drugs such as psilocybin, mescaline, and MDA (methylenedioxyamphetamine). I have also observed many hundreds of people under the influence of these substances. Along with the mental and emotional states released by these drugs, I have experienced and observed some remarkable objective changes in body function that are very pertinent to the subject of mind-body relations and should be of great interest to medical researchers and practitioners. Two kinds of changes particularly fascinate me: disappearance of allergies and appearance of "supernormal" abilities to tolerate strong stimulation.

I have seen many cases of complete loss of allergic response in people under the influence of psychedelic drugs. For example, I once watched a man with a lifelong cat allergy play with a cat several hours after taking a dose of LSD in a setting that encouraged deep and blissful relaxation. He was with a small group of friends, all in similar euphoric states. Their emotional support helped him feel totally nondefensive and at one with the people, animals, and plants in a beautiful garden. When a cat walked up to him, he began to handle it without thinking of the consequences. Ordinarily, he got an intense reaction within minutes of touching any cat: itching and swelling of his eyes and upper respiratory membranes, sneezing, and hives on any area of skin licked by the animal. Now, for the first time he could remember, nothing untoward happened. He took pleasure in caressing and stroking the cat and in receiving its attentions.

Although the absence of an allergic reaction impressed him greatly, he said it seemed natural and unsurprising, given how he was feeling about himself and the cat. Several days later, not under the influence of any drug, he tried petting another cat and did react, although somewhat less violently than usual. The experience on LSD made him believe in the possibility of being free of this problem and showed him it had some relationship to his state of mind and body, not just to the presence of a cat. That realization motivated him to look for ways of controlling his allergies other than by avoiding allergens or taking antihistamines, which suppressed his symptoms but always made him groggy and depressed.

While in this same kind of psychedelic state, I have noticed that I do not react to insect bites. Instead of the usual itching welts, I have nothing to show but tiny red dots that cause no discomfort. Sometimes, when the drugs wear off after twelve hours or the next day, typical allergic reactions to the bites will appear. Sometimes they do not.

I have also observed complete disappearance of hay fever and allergic asthma in users of psychedelics, even when those conditions have been intense, persistent, and ongoing at the time of taking the drug. Again, the effect is usually temporary, but sometimes when the conditions reappear, they are muted.

I have had little success in persuading researchers to examine this phenomenon. Some pharmacologists have listened to my stories, then replied, "Well, of course, that's only to be expected. LSD and the other psychedelics are all stimulants that produce adrenergic states; the release of adrenaline explains any suppression of allergic responsiveness." In other words, most pharmacologists refuse to see anything extraordinary in these experiences and are not going to pay any more attention to them.

It is true that psychedelics affect the adrenaline system of the body and that adrenaline blocks allergic reactions. (An injection of adrenaline is the standard emergency treatment for life-threatening allergic shock.) That cannot be the whole story, however, because just having psychedelics and stimulants in your body does not automatically make allergies go away. You have to be in a particular state of relaxed, blissful, nondefensive openness. People having bad trips on LSD, who are paranoid, withdrawn, and sure they are dying or losing their minds, do not show this effect, even though they are in adrenergic states.

Furthermore, the fact of correlation between mental state and allergy is hardly obscure. Many people, both patients and doctors, are aware of it. What is impressive in these psychedelic experiences is how quickly and completely allergies dematerialize when people are truly relaxed and content. It is those states of mind that are key. Undoubtedly, there are many roads to them. Psychedelics make them accessible only under proper conditions of set and setting but might be useful in teaching people how it feels to be free of allergic reactions.

I can envision a training program in which patients would have weekly psychedelic sessions in optimal settings after careful preparation to motivate them to control their allergies. At the start the pills would contain full doses of drugs, but each week the dose would be reduced until the pill was just an inactive placebo, and the patients would be doing it all on their own. Then they would have to practice creating the desired state outside of the training facility, especially in real-world situations likely to provoke their allergies.

That allergies can vanish totally in certain mental states is reason to explore the connections between the mind and the immune system, since allergy represents unbalanced functioning of that system.

An even more dramatic experience on psychedelic drugs is the appearance of supernormal abilities to interact safely with normally injurious objects and forces.

In 1970 I took LSD with a group of friends on a perfect spring day at my house in rural Virginia. After adjusting to the physical and perceptual changes caused by the drug, I felt elated, full of energy and confidence, and delightfully limber. Around the house were several walkways covered with crushed rocks. Ordinarily, I could not walk on these barefoot. After a few steps, the pain would be too much for me, and the sharp stones would leave indentations on my tender soles. Now I found myself walking barefoot on these same stones with impunity. Not only did they not hurt me, they felt good. I wiggled my feet into them, danced over them, and jumped up and down on them. None of this left any marks on my feet. I was astonished at my ability, also delighted. Next day, I tried to repeat it but could not. The stones hurt and left the usual marks.

I have since had other experiences of this sort, at first only under the influence of psychedelics but later without them. Also, I have seen others experiment in similar ways and discover similar abilities. These include: (1) the ability to handle rough or sharp objects, such as spiny cactuses, without being scratched or hurt; (2) the ability to receive repeated and forceful blows without sustaining injury or even marks on the skin; (3) the ability to tolerate cold water or cold air without clothing, yet remain warm and feel warm to the touch of other people; (4) the ability to touch and walk upon surfaces so hot they are intolerable to others and quickly cause burns.

If I had not experienced these abilities myself and seen them in others, I might not believe them possible. Knowing them to be real, I am eager to find out what they represent and how to work with them.

There are two aspects to all of these experiences: a subjective change in sensitivity to pain and discomfort, and an objective change in bodily response to strong stimulation. The first is easy to explain. The second is not easy to explain and is also more important.

Most people know that subjective tolerance for pain varies with circumstances. A slap that would be intensely painful if given in anger can be easily tolerated if given in friendly play. We now have endorphins to explain changes in pain tolerance as well. Also, psychiatrists have long known that awareness of pain can be completely suppressed in states of "hysterical dissociation" — the "shock" that comes over victims of devastating accidents and wounded soldiers on battlefields. In dissociated states, pain signals from the injured body are denied access to consciousness, probably a protective reaction enabling injured persons to maintain enough awareness to seek help or safety. Such persons do not look or act normal. They may stare fixedly, be unresponsive to questions, and not fully be aware of their surroundings.

When people in psychedelic states experience the supernormal abilities described above, they tend to be relaxed, calm, and fully aware of their surroundings and bodies. Most important, their bodies are reacting to stress in a different way, not just feeling different. A walk on sharp stones does not hurt, but it also leaves no marks on the feet. Not only does handling a hot object cause no discomfort, it causes no burns. It is this objective component of the change that is so remarkable. Neither endorphins nor psychiatry can explain it, and it cries out for explanation.

I can only speculate about these abilities in the absence of any research on them. As with the disappearance of allergies, it is a distinctive mental state that seems responsible, not the psychedelics. No drug will confer these abilities automatically, but once experienced, they can be re-created without the drugs. Even more impressive forms of them appear in other cultures where no drugs are used to acquire them. (I will discuss fire walking as an example in a moment.)

One of the chief aspects of the psychosomatic state that allows the body to absorb unusually strong stimulation without injury is relaxation — complete and balanced relaxation leaving muscles free of imposed tension. Most people stand, sit, lie, and move with their muscles held in patterns of learned tension that develop over lifetimes and are unconscious and unnoticed because they are always present. Many systems of psychotherapy and body work agree that painful experiences, emotions, and memories can find their way to the musculature and simply remain there as frozen patterns of energy.[4] Nerves and muscles live in intimate balance, so that the state of the muscles reflects the state of the nervous system. I am sure that neuromuscular activity is one major expression of mind-body interaction.

Possibly, our muscles are capable of remarkable feats when

they are freed from mental interference conveyed to them by nerves. If the muscles in the foot are totally free, perhaps they can react to pressure with precise responses that neutralize even very strong forces. Step on a sharp rock, and the muscle receiving the impact might be able to press back in just the right place and with just enough pressure to balance it. There would then be no net force on the skin and no indentation to see afterward.

It feels to me as if this is the sort of mechanism at work in some of the experiences described earlier. The secret of withstanding forceful blows is not to anticipate pain or to try to defend against them. Anticipation and defense translate into tension, and tense muscles cannot interact freely with external objects and forces. It is then that pain and injury result. Again, the key is in the mind, because it is the mind, acting through nerves, that allows or prevents free responsiveness of muscles. If my sense of this process is right, there is great value in learning to relax, not in the usual, superficial ways, but in the profound way that reveals our true capacities and strengths. I am sure these "supernormal" abilities are quite natural and ought to be normal. We just do not give ourselves enough chances to experience them.

Relaxation and precise muscular responsiveness can account for some of the abilities I have mentioned but not others. They do not explain how people can tolerate extremes of heat and cold. In those cases, other mechanisms must be at work.

Fire Walking

Walking barefoot on beds of red-hot coals or glowing rocks is a common practice in many parts of the world, especially the Orient. Often fire walking is performed as a religious ritual in large public ceremonies.

In Japan, walks on hot coals take place at Buddhist temples on a particular festival day. After processions of monks make the walk, ordinary people, women and children included, take off their sandals and follow them over the coals. These Japanese fire walkers recite silently a certain Buddhist prayer and say they do not get burned if they keep their minds on it.

In Singapore, fire walking is the highlight of a week-long

annual festival at a major Hindu temple. There the fire pit is awesomely large and hot. The festival honors a goddess who is known to grant the petitions and prayers of the faithful. They undertake the walk as proof of their devotion to her, believing that if their faith is pure, she will transform the burning coals to flowers beneath their feet. Of the hundreds of participants, a very few are badly burned each year, but these calamities are considered essential to the festival because they demonstrate the injurious potential of the fire pit and the miraculous nature of successful walks across it.

In some island cultures of the South Pacific, fire walking is done over red-hot rocks, which are much hotter than coals. The walkers work themselves into states of expectant excitement and concentration by means of dancing, drumming, and chanting. A master of ceremonies, expert in the practice, judges when a man is ready to face the ordeal, and under his direction, most people come through the walk unharmed.

In Sri Lanka, fire walkers prepare for their performance by a week or two of fasting, prayer, meditation, bathing, chanting, and sexual abstinence. They say anyone can walk on fire who practices these acts of devotion and austerity.

Some Europeans walk on fire, mainly in Spain, Bulgaria, and Greece. Many tourists come to watch the fire walkers of the Greek village of Ayia Eleni when they perform at the annual festival honoring saints Constantine and Helen. The villagers run, dance, walk, and hop through an enormous bed of glowing coals, all the while shouting and holding aloft sacred icons. These men and women believe Saint Constantine's power protects them from injury. The same power, they say, cures them of illnesses and enables them to cure others.

In the United States, some members of the splinter Christian sects that handle poisonous snakes to show their faith also handle fire, directing flames from kerosene torches on their bare hands and faces without experiencing injury.

The fact of fire walking is not in dispute. Too many people have witnessed it, and too many careful observers have recorded detailed accounts of it. What is in contention is the interpretation to be placed on it. I am sorry to say the scientific literature on fire walking is dreadful. What few good articles it contains are the work of anthropologists. Hardly any physiologists or medical scientists have studied the phenomenon, and those who have written about it have mostly tried to make it appear unremarkable. Their aim is to defuse the challenge it poses to the materialistic conception of the human organism. Some of these people have actually said in print that the whole explanation lies in Asians' having tough feet and a high tolerance for pain. Others have called fire walking a trick and stated their refusal to be taken in by crafty natives. The exact nature of the trick is never revealed, though a few articles speculate about mysterious salves that fire walkers apply surreptitiously to their feet to prevent burns. (Of course, no known substance has such an effect.)

Recently, as reports of fire walking have grown more numerous and drawn more attention, some scientists have advanced a more sophisticated mechanistic theory. They say a microlayer of air, formed by evaporation of sweat, can efficiently insulate the sole of the foot from the heat of red-hot coals. This is a known physical effect; it explains why a drop of water flicked into a very hot skillet can retain its integrity and dance about for some time without boiling off. The appeal of this theory for the scientists who propose it is its avoidance of any reference to the mind or the power of consciousness to modify physical reality.

This mechanism might play a part in walks over hot coals, but it cannot explain how some fire walkers shuffle leisurely through ankle-deep layers of red-hot cinders or walk over glowing rocks at temperatures much too high for microlayers of air to afford protection to the skin. In 1974, a nuclear physicist from the Max Planck Institute for Plasma Physics in Munich made careful measurements of the temperatures of rocks in a Fijian fire pit and of the feet of the fire walkers. The rocks were over 600 degrees Fahrenheit, but the feet never got hotter than 150 degrees. The physicist noted that a piece of calloused skin from one of the native's feet carbonized almost instantly when it was placed on a rock. He concluded that whatever was happening was not explainable within the realm of known physics.[5]

Some fire walkers say their feet feel cold during the event. Others say they feel warmth or electric tingling. A few report strong sensations of heat. Some walk the coals in religious ecstasies or trances, but others do it in simple states of expectant concentration. All say fire walking allows them to transcend their ordinary limitations and has great personal meaning. Given my own experiences and observations of related abilities during psychedelic states, I am inclined to regard fire walking as another example of an extraordinary capacity of the body, unmasked during certain states of consciousness. I have no doubt that physical mechanisms mediate it, but I am sure they involve the nervous system and are under the control of mind.

Several different mechanisms may take part. Changes in blood circulation might help conduct heat away from body surfaces or reduce flow of heat to vulnerable tissues. Changes in the functions of local nerves might suppress the activity of neurochemicals that mediate pain and inflammatory reaction to strong stimulation, especially since experiments with hypnosis show these functions to be susceptible to modification by suggestion. A more hypothetical possibility is some as-yet-undiscovered capacity of the nervous system to absorb potentially harmful forms of energy, transform them, and conduct them away from the body surface.

Many fire walkers believe that supernatural deities and forces give them their spectacular abilities. I respect their belief and admit its practical value. Personally, I think the abilities are quite natural, the results of using the mind in certain ways (or not using it in ordinary ways) and so allowing the brain and nerves to alter the body's responsiveness to heat. I agree with the fire walkers of Greece that the power that protects them from burns can also cure disease. The mind holds the key to healing, and healing is as extraordinary as fire walking. It may also make use of some of the same nervous pathways and mechanisms. Both deserve the full attention of medical scientists who are willing to grant the importance of consciousness.

I hope I have sketched a clear picture of the power of the mind over the physical body. It can make warts go away, endow sugar pills with all the effects of strong drugs, enable medical treatments to unblock healing and produce cures of illness (or prevent them from doing so), initiate complete remissions of cancer, modify the activity of the immune system, control neurochemistry, change the body's responsiveness to environmental stimulation, affect (for better or worse) all the organs of the body regulated by the autonomic nervous system, and, I suspect, do much more.

Yet a curious theme runs through all these examples and cases: a kind of indirectness or roundaboutness of mind-body interactions. Why can't we just will our blood pressure to go down, our warts to fall off, our immune systems to mop up cancers? Why do sick people need to externalize belief to reap its benefits — to place it in healers, miracle shrines, drugs, and knives in order to let healing occur? Why do people have to take psychedelic drugs to see that allergies are totally subject to mental states? Why do fire walkers from Fiji to Greece think their powers come from deities and saints rather than from their own minds?

The answer to all these questions has to do with the nature of will and its relationship to the brain. Evidently, the part of the mind containing the will is not the part that connects directly to the nervous centers controlling these psychosomatic events.

Scientific knowledge of the human brain is very primitive. That organ is still the "great ravelled knot," in the words of one of its foremost modern investigators.* We know much more about the function of the peripheral nerves than we do of the central nervous system (brain and spinal cord), and just do not have the information to answer interesting questions about how mind and brain interact. Since the methods of science are designed to study physical objects and forces, we know even less about the mind.

In the materialistic conception of human beings, consciousness is an epiphenomenon — that is, something incidental and secondary that just happens to arise from the physical circuitry of the brain. The brain is primary, mind secondary. Therefore, mind cannot exist without an integral brain or have any reality apart from the brain. At the moment, this conception dominates the neurosciences and strongly influences medical research and practice.

That consciousness depends on brain activity is obvious. Hit a person hard enough on the head, and consciousness will be lost. Give enough of a drug that depresses brain activity (any of

*Sir Charles Sherrington (1861–1952), Nobel laureate.

the sedatives and general anesthetics), and consciousness will be lost. An overactive thyroid can produce dramatic changes of mood and behavior, including a kind of manic psychosis. A few millionths of a gram of LSD, a scarcely visible amount of the pure drug, can precipitate people into states of overwhelming bliss or terror. Direct electrical stimulation of the brain with tiny needles can give conscious surgical patients hallucinations that seem as real to them as anything going on in the operating room; it can also make them move or speak, arouse them sexually or instantly put them into states of extreme emotion, and cause them to relive past experiences. The effects last only while electrical stimulation is maintained, evaporating when it ends.

One of the pioneers of this type of brain research was the neurosurgeon Wilder Penfield (1891–1978). He took advantage of many operations to stimulate the exposed brains of patients, recording their responses and mapping areas of the brain responsible for particular sensory, emotional, and motor activities. Penfield was a committed mechanist whose experiments certainly supported the view that brain is primary and mind secondary. Yet his last book, published shortly before his death, was a philosophical exploration titled *The Mystery of the Mind*.[6] In it he came to a most unorthodox conclusion: that mind is not coextensive with brain. Some of it, he decided, exists apart from the brain and can function independent of it.

That viewpoint is popular with many other people, from yogis to Christian Scientists. I once heard a Hindu swami who demonstrated great voluntary control over his heart tell an audience of scientists that "all of the brain is concerned with the mind, but not all of the mind is in the brain." This model sees consciousness as primary, able to direct and organize brain activity and through it control the entire body. In Mary Baker Eddy's words, "Mind governs the body, not partially but wholly." Of course, Christian Science goes further by according mind greater reality than the physical body and denying that matter can limit or modify consciousness.

Wilder Penfield was much more cautious in arguing for the independence of mind from brain, but his philosophical reversal was dramatic enough to upset his colleagues. Some of them wrote it off as a manifestation of senility or of a tendency to irrationality that comes over people approaching death who cannot bear the thought of total extinction of consciousness. I find Penfield's final argument very useful, because it shows that the obvious dependence of consciousness on the activity of the brain does not automatically make it an unimportant epiphenomenon or exclude the possibility that mind can direct the brain.

Choosing between the extreme versions of these models is a question of religion and philosophy. They are, after all, only models. Maybe it is not even necessary to make an either-or choice between them, especially in their more moderate forms, because both might have their uses. Assuming that consciousness is a product of brain activity allows neuroscientists to investigate the biological basis of behavior, the actions of mind-altering drugs, and the power of endorphins and other neurochemicals to modify experience. Assuming that consciousness directs brain function and can control physiology explains many of the observations presented in this book and opens up new vistas for medicine of the twenty-first century. The first model has been well worked. I think more use of the second in the medical sciences would greatly extend our abilities to maintain health and treat disease.

A parallel situation holds for the relationship between the brain and the rest of the body. Clearly, the life of the brain depends on the life of the body. Stoppage of the heart for more than a few minutes results in irreversible brain damage. A sudden drop in blood sugar is also a disaster for brain cells; they need constant supplies of glucose, the only nutrient they can use. At the same time, a strong case can be made for the brain as the reason for the existence of the body, since every system is directly concerned with maintaining or protecting the life of the central nervous system (or reproducing it in a new organism). In a developing embryo it is the nervous system that organizes the structures of the future body. Every organ, every cell of a human being is linked and held in service to the brain by the endless branching of the peripheral nerves.

Human consciousness, particularly ego consciousness associated with verbal thought and will, seems related to the activity of the cerebral cortex, the thin layer of cells that covers the two hemispheres of the brain. The control centers of normally involuntary functions, of the endocrine glands and the immune system, of placebo responses and innate healing, seem to be located far from the cortex in deep, midline structures, such as the evolutionarily old brainstem, which connects the hemispheres to the spinal cord. These centers certainly respond to some suggestions and beliefs but not to purely cortical beliefs and voluntary commands. There appears to be some barrier to direct transmission of conscious thought from the cortex to the deep centers controlling the mechanisms of psychosomatic events, including healing.

Whatever that barrier is — and it may be a long time before neuroscientists discover its nature — it necessitates roundabout ways of putting will and belief into bodily action; hence the strange and varied forms of medical treatment, the curiosities of placebos, the need to project belief onto external objects, substances, people, and gods in order to draw on its power.

I have written a lot about the power of belief in these pages, but I now must distinguish between superficial belief and belief that counts. If you believe it will rain today because you heard a forecast of rain on the radio, that is superficial belief. If you believe it will rain today because an arthritic joint has started to ache in a way you have learned to associate with approaching rain, that is belief that counts. If I believe a shaman has power over me because I have an intellectual interest in shamanism, that is not the same as believing it because I have seen him produce unexplainable effects and feel physical fear in his presence. Christian Scientists make good patients because they bring real belief to medical situations. When they are forced to seek help from doctors, their strong feelings about breaking a fundamental prohibition of their religion give added power to any drugs they take.

Belief that counts is gut-level belief that stirs emotions and connects to the body through the centers of the deep brain. It is based on experience as well as thought and must be psychosomatic to begin with, bridging the barrier between modern cortex and primitive brainstem.

This necessity is cause for both hope and despair. It means people cannot just will themselves to be healthy or set their innate healing mechanisms in motion whenever needed. It also means they are not likely to be conscious of the ways they now block healing, stress their bodies, and create susceptibility to external agents of disease by sending negative mental energies through those same mechanisms. The requirement that belief must penetrate to levels of mind and brain below ordinary consciousness in order to work its magic makes it unlikely that people will ever be free of the need for substances, treatments, doctors, and deities.

On the other hand, understanding the power of belief and the mind to modify the body in good ways should make people much more aware of their own potentials to deal with illness and adversity, whether or not they can realize them by acts of will. It should also motivate both doctors and patients to find better, safer methods of allowing healing to occur, such as the use of active drugs that evoke placebo responses but cause fewer adverse reactions than those now in favor. Research on new psychosomatic therapies has already produced techniques such as biofeedback and systems of relaxation and visualization that really change physiological problems for the better. I expect to see more of them.

Research on the specifics of mind-body communication will be the frontier of medicine in the twenty-first century. I would be very surprised if it did not result in ideas and methods to help people take more responsibility for their own health, encourage them to practice true preventive medicine on their own, and prepare them to make intelligent choices of practitioners and treatments when they need outside help. The overall result will be a healthier society.

VI

HEALTH AND HEALING IN THE YEAR 2000

22

What Doctors Can Learn from Physicists

REGULAR MEDICINE of the current century views the human organism as a complicated mechanism. It minimizes or ignores consciousness and mind as important determinants of health, illness, and responses to treatments. Regular medicine also likes to call itself scientific and imagines that its exclusive attention to the physical reality of bodily mechanisms is in the best spirit of twentieth-century science. What most medical doctors do not know is that the scientific model of reality has changed radically since 1900 and no longer views the universe as an orderly mechanism independent of the consciousness observing it.

Doctors may find it useful to act like scientists for many reasons, not least because it enables them to draw on the great belief of patients today in science and technology. Nonetheless, medicine can never be a science like physics or chemistry because health and illness are so close to the mysteries at the heart of existence.

Science is an intellectual method of gaining knowledge; the very word comes from the Latin verb *scire*, "to know," and intellect can never explain away ultimate mysteries. At best it can approach them by describing the details of their outward manifestations. Of course, gravity, light, chemical combustion, and nuclear fusion are also expressions of deep mysteries, but physicists and chemists can keep themselves usefully busy by looking for better and better interpretations of those forces and interactions, thereby rolling back the frontiers of the unknown. The practical urgencies of illness do not permit the luxury of scientific contemplation. They demand immediate action. Doctors must deal head-on with the mystery of good and evil, the mystery of

HEALTH AND HEALING

balance, the mystery of mind and body, the mystery of death. Although medical science can help by clarifying the body's structure and function, the healing art will remain an art.

"Scientific medicine" is not very old — less than a century — and its view of reality is frozen in an obsolete mold. I would like to see medicine become more scientific in its theory while acknowledging the artful, magical, and religious nature of its practice.

The specific goals of science are to increase our ability to describe, predict, and control the phenomenal world. When it succeeds, science gives us power as well as knowledge, power to use the forces of nature. Joseph Priestly's experiments on "dephlogisticated air" in 1774 enabled the great French chemist Lavoisier (1743–1794) to discover oxygen and propose a new theory of combustion. His explanation that combustion represented chemical combination of a burning substance with oxygen made better sense than any previous theory. It allowed him to understand how plants and animals get energy from foods and later allowed inventors to build the internal combustion engines that have transformed the world.

In addition to giving us understanding and power, scientific success provides emotional comfort. The human intellect fears unpredictability and impotence in the face of a mysterious, possibly hostile universe. Primitive peoples whose astronomical science was unable to predict eclipses of the sun must have felt sheer terror when the source of life suddenly and unaccountably went out, especially if no one in a tribe or village had lived through such an event before. The success of our astronomical model of the solar system in describing and predicting eclipses is one example of the way science can be comforting by reducing primitive fears based on ignorance.

Scientists try to make sense of observed phenomena, to find patterns and regularities that make for better descriptions, fewer surprises, and greater control. How well they succeed depends on the theoretical models they use. Theories are the pictures scientists construct of reality, through which they interpret their observations. These pictures change as science evolves. New theories may originate in intuitive flashes (like the one about gravity triggered by Isaac Newton's falling apple), or they may be suggested by results of experiments differing from the predictions of existing models (like Einstein's special theory of relativity). New theories are better or worse only insofar as they further or impede the basic scientific goals of description, prediction, and control.

Enlightened scientists never forget that theories are pictures of reality, not reality itself — the maps, not the territory. Albert Einstein wrote in 1938:

> In our endeavor to understand reality we are somewhat like a man trying to understand the mechanism of a closed watch. He sees the face and the moving hands, even hears its ticking, but he has no way of opening the case. If he is ingenious, he may form some picture of a mechanism which could be responsible for all the things he observes, but he may never be quite sure his picture is the only one which could explain his observations. He will never be able to compare his picture with the real mechanism and he cannot even imagine the possibility of the meaning of such a comparison.[1]

For the rest of us, the distinction between theory and reality is easy to forget, especially when a popular theory accords with our common-sense experience and so seems "right." The chemical model that interprets combustion as the combination of fuel molecules with oxygen works very well, but it is only a model. No one can prove that a better and different one will never come along. This is the limitation of science as an intellectual pursuit: it cannot reveal ultimate truth, just come up with better and better approximations of it in the form of theoretical models.

Mystics claim to be able to perceive reality directly by means other than the intellect — to open the case of Einstein's watch and look inside. They say direct experience of the deep mysteries is ultimately comforting, but unfortunately, they cannot communicate it to others. The limitation of scientific knowledge is offset by the ease of communicating it and putting it to use throughout society. Mystics, if they talk at all, try to convey their intensely personal visions in songs, poems, and indirect analogies. Those efforts may inspire people to follow in their path but do not let others know what they know. A mathematical statement of a scientific law allows one investigator to communicate directly with another and the two of them to work together at clarifying the nature of reality. By constructing and testing better theoretical approximations of the truth, scientists gain understanding and power that can be shared and used by all people.

The history of science is an endless saga of theoretical revolution. New theories usually appear suddenly and rarely meet with immediate or universal acceptance, even if they confer descriptive and predictive advantage. Commonly, their first proponents find themselves in conflict with the orthodoxy of the day and even with the public at large, especially if prevailing theories seem adequate and appeal to emotional needs. The Copernican model of the solar system with the sun at its center met such resistance because the old picture with the earth at the center was consistent with common sense and also gratified desires to see humanity as the central focus of the cosmos.

Regular medicine's denial of consciousness as a determinant of health and healing seemed right in the late 1800s when allopaths decided to become scientists. In those days the prevailing scientific theory had no place for human consciousness. It was an elaborate development of a picture of reality drawn by Sir Isaac Newton (1642–1727) two hundred years earlier, which described matter and energy as quantities independent of the mind describing them. In the Newtonian model the universe was an orderly mechanism that went lawfully about its business whether or not anyone was looking at it. Physicists have long since rejected it in favor of a better model, but most medical doctors are unaware of the implications of the change for their field.

Newton's picture was (and is) very appealing. It demystified much of reality, putting distance between the modern, scientific world and a superstitious past in which people lived in fear of supernatural forces and unpredictable deities. Also, it worked very well, conferring a high degree of ability to describe, predict, and control the observable world. Electricity and magnetism were unavailable for human use until so recently because people had no theoretical model to make sense of them before Newton's work provided one. Using his model, Western scientists were able to achieve an unprecedented level of technological power in the 1800s and thus dominate the world. By the turn of the last century, Newtonian theory was able to explain most physical phenomena then observable, leaving few anomalies unexplained. Disaffected theorists had little incentive to try to come up with any better picture of the nature of space, time, matter, and energy.

Speaking to the Royal Institution in 1900, the British physicist and inventor Lord Kelvin (1824–1907) noted only two "clouds" on the horizon of physics and expressed confidence that they, too, would soon dissolve in the light of reason working within the framework of established theory.[2] He could not have been more wrong.

One of Lord Kelvin's clouds was the problem of black-body radiation: why atoms appear to absorb and emit energy in discrete spurts rather than in a smooth and continuous fashion. It led conservative German physicist Max Planck in December of 1900 to formulate the first part of a new physical theory — quantum theory — that was destined to overthrow Newtonian mechanics before very long. Planck never intended that result; he just wanted to find an explanation for an anomaly unaccounted for by the accepted model of the atom, but the anomaly proved to be an expression of a major defect in Newtonian theory, and the explanation turned out to be the seed of a new and very different picture of physical reality.

The other cloud on Lord Kelvin's horizon was the Michelson-Morley experiment of 1887, which disproved the existence of an "ether" — the tenuous physical medium that light was supposed to travel through. That result indicated an unexpected property of light and led Einstein in 1905 to formulate his special theory of relativity. In it he rewrote Newton's laws of motion. Relativity theory undermined the foundations of the Newtonian model from another direction and with quantum theory ushered in the new physics of the twentieth century.

With the overthrow of the old model, the observing mind entered physical theory in ways that would have scandalized orthodox physicists of the 1800s. For example, Einstein's theory showed that mass and time were not absolute but relative to the observer's state of motion. Quantum theory demonstrated that what can be known about atomic particles depends on what observers choose to measure: if you want to be certain about an electron's position in space, you cannot know its momentum, and vice versa. Suddenly, physical quantities were no longer independent of the minds of scientists, and these early suggestions of the interdependence of external reality and consciousness were to develop into later theories that would have scandalized Planck and Einstein.

The new physics quickly brought about dramatic jumps in understanding and control. Because of it scientists can make sense of many of their observations of stars and galaxies and can harness forces in the atom much more powerful than any previously available for human use. Also, it holds out the promise of even greater advances, such as the possibility of explaining the basic forces of the universe as different expressions of one fundamental interaction.[3]

Along with bits of the new model, students of physics today still learn Newton's laws of motion and many other theories that would be perfectly familiar to scientists of the last century. The reason is that Newtonian mechanics is easy to teach and works to explain observations of the ordinary world of the five senses. Only at velocities near the speed of light do the effects of special relativity invalidate the predictions of Newtonian mechanics; at ordinary velocities the discrepancies are so small that Newton's laws serve as good approximations. Only on the scale of individual atoms and electrons do the predictions of quantum theory contradict the predictions of common sense. It is not that the old model was wrong, but that the new one is better. It has greater explanatory power, especially when we extend our powers of observation to the galactic and atomic scales by means of instruments.

Einstein used a good simile to describe this relationship between old and new theories:

> . . . creating a new theory is not like destroying an old barn and erecting a skyscraper in its place. It is rather like climbing a mountain, gaining new and wider views, discovering unexpected connections between our starting point and its rich environment. But the point from which we started still exists and can be seen, although it appears smaller and forms a tiny part of our broad view gained by the mastery of the obstacles on our adventurous way up.[4]

Although we can go on acting as if the old physics is an accurate picture of reality, it is not. Even if it seems consistent with our everyday experience of light and motion, it may get us in trouble elsewhere by limiting our ability to describe, predict, and control other important phenomena.

If you are not a physicist, however, trying to get the new picture is not easy. The principles of contemporary physics are stated in mathematical formulations not easily translatable into ordinary language. They do not conjure up recognizable images or make straightforward connections with everyday experience. Worse, the images they do convey seem at odds with common sense.

Einstein once dismissed common sense as "nothing more than a deposit of prejudices laid down in the mind prior to the age of eighteen"[5] and was quite willing to pursue theoretical paths that led away from it. I would be reluctant to make such a generalization, since some of what we know by common sense seems both true and useful. For example, the notion that "an ounce of prevention is worth a pound of cure" accurately describes the relative difficulty of making a medical (or other) problem go away once it develops compared to the relative ease of anticipating it and acting to keep it from developing.

Physical theory has deviated so much from common-sense experience because it is mostly concerned with objects and forces not observable by the unaided senses. It deals with strange realms; therefore, the pictures of reality it draws will seem strange at first. Nonetheless, they must be reconcilable with human experience. The Copernican view of the solar system must have looked very strange when it was new and seemed to contradict the common-sense perception that all heavenly bodies revolve around the earth, but today, with our greater understanding and experience (including that of flying in jet planes halfway around the earth in a matter of hours), the idea that the earth goes around the sun seems perfectly logical.

The concept that physical phenomena cannot be separated from the consciousness observing them may provide a point of correspondence between the new model and the world of human experience. A number of commentators see striking parallels between Hindu and Buddhist conceptions of reality and those of contemporary physics.[6] Hinduism and Buddhism are grounded in experience and also assign central importance to consciousness as the ultimate "stuff" of the universe.

The early demonstrations of quantum and relativity theory of the interdependence of observer and observed have not only survived many experimental tests, they have developed into ideas that sound like the fantasies of science-fiction writers. Physicists now speculate that decisions about how to observe and measure reality actively create and shape it, bringing events from states of virtual or potential existence into actual manifestation — a far cry from the old Newtonian view of an external reality completely independent of mind. Orthodox science today is willing to consider consciousness as an active agent in the formation of reality, inseparable from it.[7]

Isaac Newton would probably not have been bothered by that speculation. The man who built the foundations of the model of the universe that held sway until the twentieth century was deeply religious and of mystical bent. The world remembers him for work he completed while still a young man, but he spent the rest of his long life trying to reconcile astrology and astronomy, decipher occult truths from mathematical symbols, and demonstrate the divine nature of creation. The very scientists who owed so much to him ignored all of his later writings as unintelligible ravings; to this day the work of the mature Newton remains largely unknown.

Why did Newton's followers come to regard belief in interaction of mind and matter as heresy? Especially during the golden age of nineteenth-century science and technology, champions of scientific orthodoxy saw it as their duty to combat superstitious thinking wherever it lurked, and they denounced that belief as flagrant superstition.

I think the answer has to do with the image scientists had of themselves a hundred years ago. They saw their work as an alternative to religion and magic, not as a complementary activity, and saw themselves as saviors of a race long held in bondage by ignorance and superstition. The basic premise of magic is that macrocosm and microcosm are linked, that external and internal reality are interdependent. By understanding that relationship, the magician tries to change reality through operations of the mind. The same premise underlies religious practices: what else is prayer, after all? It also occurs in many of the alternative medical systems I have reviewed. In fact, their emphasis on changes in consciousness as keys to health and healing gives them the occasional advantage over regular medicine, even when the rest of their theories are inconsistent with scientific fact.

The aversion scientists of the last century had toward admitting consciousness into their model of the universe probably was rooted in their sense of its importance to magicians, mystics, faith healers, and other people with whom they did not wish to associate. Scientific ignorance of the nature of consciousness and awareness of the mystery in it must also have contributed to that attitude, for if scientists hope to gain credibility by reducing fears of the unknown, they cannot afford to confront the unexplainable. Then, as now, mind was an ultimate mystery. Keeping it strictly separate from matter must have seemed desirable. As faith in science mounted in the Western world, its defenders made that separation an article of their faith and laxity about maintaining it grounds for expulsion from the scientific community.

Orthodox medicine decided to wed itself to science and technology at the end of the nineteenth century, just when the old model and its accompanying dogma were at the peak of their influence. As a supplicant at the temple of science, the medical profession must have been aware that it would be carefully scrutinized for signs of superstitious thinking and practice. It must also have been embarrassed about its recent past.

Remember that the Age of Heroic Medicine extended to the middle 1800s. The bleedings and purgings of that era had no basis in scientific experiment and caused such harm that the public turned against doctors and tried to strip them of political power. European and American physicians did not repudiate those practices until about 1860. Then they switched to dispensing vast quantities of opiates and alcohol (and later, cocaine), drugs that affected patients' moods without altering underlying pathology. The widespread addiction that resulted again outraged the public and created renewed interest in rival systems of treatment. For much of the second half of the nineteenth century, the regular profession was caught up in bitter struggles against homeopaths, osteopaths, Christian Scientists, and other competitors whose appeal lay in their use of methods that did not kill or cause worse suffering than the diseases they were meant to treat.

The decision to become scientific saved the embattled medical profession. With a zeal fueled by self-doubt, doctors embraced the reigning theoretical model and the attitudes that went with it. They disowned the medical practices of the past and resolved to bring professional medicine into the twentieth century as a true science, not as an art, religion, or form of magic.

Courses in physics, chemistry, and biology became the foundation of a new kind of medical education. The scientific method of controlled observation and experiment provided the means to analyze the phenomena of health and illness and evaluate treatments. Medical applications of technology produced inventions such as X-ray photography and synthetic drugs that greatly increased the power of physicians to diagnose disease and modify the structure and function of the human body. As scientists, doctors could denigrate the competition with more authority. They could prove the worthlessness of Hahnemann's theory by pointing out its incompatibility with the facts of chemistry. They could dismiss the teachings of Mary Baker Eddy and Andrew Taylor Still as unscientific because of frequent references to superstitious concepts like "mind," "God," and "the healing power of nature" that had no basis in scientific theory. Moreover, in their new role, doctors were able to take advantage of the public's growing faith in science to regain lost prestige. They must also have become better at eliciting healing responses grounded in belief. Becoming scientific was the most successful course organized medicine ever took. Within fifty years it made the profession dominant in the West and most of the rest of the world as well.

Ironically, at the very time that regular doctors began to ape the behavior and styles of physical scientists, physics began to undergo the turbulent theoretical revolution that produced a new model of reality with consciousness at its heart. Even as professional medical organizations drew up their guidelines for scientific curriculums and forced old-fashioned and rival schools to close, and even as the first breakthroughs of the new science of medicine began to convince an enthralled public that this century would see the triumph of technology over disease, the model of reality that doctors took as their own was obsolete.

Physics may seem a long way from medicine, but since it describes the stuff of which everything is made, it must influence all the other sciences. In the world of ordinary experience, the materialistic and mechanistic theories of the past may continue to seem right and work as reasonable approximations, but if consciousness has to be included to explain observed properties of atomic particles, it cannot be independent of systems composed of those particles, whether rocks, stars, plants, or, especially, human beings.

Yet the dramatic revolution in the thinking of physicists has not automatically changed the thinking of other scientists, many of whom still act as if mind and matter were unconnected and still feel threatened by suggestions to the contrary. Certainly the implications of the old model's overthrow have not yet penetrated the professional consciousness of regular medicine as the current century draws to a close.[8]

The disciplines we call sciences today differ greatly in exactness and rigor as well as in ability to describe, predict, and control the aspects of reality they care about. Physics is truly a "hard" science in terms of mathematical rigor and precision of method. Psychology and sociology are at an opposite extreme. They use many of the forms of hard science, including mathematics, experimentation, and statistical analysis of data, but the phenomena they study do not lend themselves to anything like the exact scrutiny that physicists can apply to the study of light, motion, and atomic interactions. Most psychologists and sociologists know that, but perhaps because theirs are young disciplines, often attacked from many quarters, they tend to be defensive and put on aggressive scientific airs. The results are sometimes amusing. Psychology — the study of the mind — is dominated today by a model called behaviorism that attempts to explain the behavior of animals and human beings without any reference to mind or consciousness.

The biological sciences lie somewhere between the extremes of physics and psychology. Biological phenomena can be described, predicted, and controlled with greater precision than human emotions or social movements but not with the exactness possible for chemical and atomic reactions. Biologists look down their noses at psychologists as unscientific and worry about hardening up their own discipline. In universities today, the old-fashioned biological specialties like botany and comparative zoology occupy small corners of departments whose laboratories bristle with the paraphernalia of physicists and chemists and whose blackboards are covered with mathematical formulas rather than Latin names.

A familiar defensiveness is visible within these departments. The chemotaxonomist, who classifies plants by study of their chemistry, looks down on the descriptive taxonomist, who relies on anatomy. Molecular geneticists have more scientific status than ecologists, but mathematical ecologists, who use statistical models to explain biological events, are catching up. Biochemists rate high in prestige, biophysicists even higher. Most of these people regard medical doctors with disdain.

The sneering of Ph.D.'s at M.D.'s for being "soft" in their science is often tinged with envy of the earning power of the medical degree. In any case, it makes physicians defensive in turn and encourages them to make greater displays of the forms of what they imagine to be hard science. The public's worship of science and technology reinforces this behavior.

Medical doctors often dismiss psychology as a pseudoscience and refer to their own colleagues in psychiatry as "witch doctors." They think it is their job to dispel magical and religious conceptions of health and disease. They welcome more and more mathematics, physics, and chemistry in medical curriculums and more technological instrumentation in hospitals. They invite patients to dream along with them that the clear light of medical science will erase all superstitions of the past, including rival systems of treatment, and with them the diseases that plague humanity — even, perhaps, death itself. They want everyone to see them as real scientists and medicine as a real science, a hard one, just like physics.

Meanwhile, physics has gone totally soft by the nineteenth-century standards doctors still use. Sooner or later, the theoretical revolution in physics will catch up with medical science. I hope the change will come sooner, because the exaggerated scientism of regular medicine is leading us in dangerous directions, as I have tried to show in the course of this book.

If health and illness are rooted in the deep mysteries and eliciting healing is an art that can draw profitably from the techniques of magic and religion, what is the place of science in medicine? I am not in any way arguing against the concept of medical science, but I do urge medical scientists to take notice of current theory of the nature of reality and to distinguish between good information and bad information.

Scientific knowledge of human biology does not automatically translate into medical practice. A lot of it is irrelevant, and some of it is misleading. Medical journals are so cluttered with useless information gained by scientific observation and experiment that finding really important facts in them takes much longer than it should. The bulk of medical science today is busywork that would be merely forgettable if it did not make the medical literature and the curriculums of medical schools so unwieldy.

Wrong information is worse than useless information. Many medical researchers try to test hypotheses that are unreasonable to begin with by shoddy experimental procedures, then draw conclusions unjustified by the methods. Because few practitioners are adept at analyzing published research with a critical eye, these misleading results may influence practice with unfortunate consequences for patients. The problem of bad research is especially common in fields contaminated by emotional bias and political tensions, such as drug abuse, sexuality, birth control, nutrition, the management of mental illness, unorthodox treatment, and so forth. Bad research in these areas crops up even in the best medical journals.*

Few articles in medical journals today seem to me to contribute much to the cause of thoughtful prevention and treatment of disease. Many of the rest look scientific in their use of technical jargon, graphs, and tables, but even the ones that draw conclu-

*For example, the wrong idea that LSD breaks chromosomes and thereby causes genetic damage first appeared in an impressive-looking article in the prestigious *New England Journal of Medicine*, which endorsed its conclusion in an accompanying editorial.[9] That was in 1967. It was a product of bad research on a highly emotional subject and received great attention by the news media. Despite its thorough disproof by good tests conducted a few years later, the error persists, and people still believe it.[10]

sions justified by their methods and data remain academic exercises uninspired by intelligence and of no therapeutic import.

Good scientific research on the mind-body can be very helpful to medical doctors. It can make them aware of the structure and function of bodily organs in ways that change practice for the better. Demonstration of the role of the thymus gland in directing cells of the immune system discredited the concept of the thymus as a useless organ and brought a swift end to the unscientific procedure of irradiating the gland to treat its "pathological enlargement" in children. Demonstration of the ability of inactive placebos to reduce anginal pain as well as or better than iproniazid spared thousands of patients with coronary insufficiency the harmful side effects of that drug. Research on the nature of DNA, genes, and genetic control of cellular activity has begun to suggest ways of modifying inherited diseases, viral infections, and cancer.

Obviously, science has much to contribute to the healing art. It is just that science must be good if it is to make for good medicine — good not only in its method but in its theory and inspiration. Medical scientists who are willing to work from sound definitions of health and healing and explore new models for making sense of illness and its treatment will be able to design research of far greater relevance to medical practice than those who are not. The whole question of how mind and body interact is practically virgin territory for scientific study. Since the interdependence of mind and matter is now firmly established in the model of reality used by contemporary physicists, medical researchers ought to have no qualms about studying it. There is no longer anything unscientific about psychosomatic phenomena. We just need information on the details and mechanisms of mind-body interactions.

If medical science will turn its attention toward that end, medical practice of the next century will be transformed, and our power to prevent and treat illness will increase as much as our technological power increased in the past hundred years.

23

New Medicine for a New Century

THE YEAR 2000 is an arbitrary date for the end of one period of history and the beginning of another.* Nevertheless, the appearance of such a new and round figure on calendars will inspire analysts to look backward and forward in efforts to summarize past developments and anticipate coming ones. The turn of the last century did prove to be a watershed in science; it coincided with the beginnings of the new physics. This one happens to be the turn of a whole millennium. I hope philosophers of the twenty-second century will be able to look back on it as the beginning of the new medicine.

In these pages I have dealt mainly with ideas rather than with techniques. I will feel I have succeeded in my purpose if readers question old assumptions about health, healing, disease, and treatment and replace them with more useful ones. Medical theories are not worth much, however, unless they give rise to practices that work. I would like to see researchers, practitioners, and patients all try to apply these ideas in their own ways.

I have already indicated the kinds of research that need to be started. Nothing more than outmoded concepts keeps scientists from trying to discover the mechanisms of wart cures, placebo responses, hypnotic induction of blisters, and the rest of the anomalous occurrences demonstrating the influence of mind on body. Nothing but lack of scientific information keeps doctors from taking greater advantage of that influence to design safer and better treatments and preventive strategies. I urge forward-

---

*Anyway, the twenty-first century does not start until January 1, 2001. The year 2000 is the last year of the present century.

looking researchers to concentrate on the anomalies of human biology, take them seriously, and go to work on them.

In recounting the history of homeopathy, I explained how Samuel Hahnemann coined the word *allopathic* ("other than the disease") to describe regular medical practice, because he thought it prescribed treatments on the basis of no logical or consistent relationship to symptoms. I mentioned also that nineteenth-century allopaths tried to disown that name and, when they failed, tried to redefine it to project a better image. They came up with a new etymology from German roots meaning "all therapies" and claimed their system embraced all methods of proven value in the treatment of disease.

Proven means "tested" — by time, by experiment, by experience. I quite like that revisionist definition. It suggests a medical practice willing to look at all systems of treatment for methods that might be useful and to try them out. I occasionally meet doctors who experiment with folk remedies and get such good results that they then design controlled experiments to convince their colleagues of the worth of the "new" procedures. I meet some doctors who are willing to try out massage and bony manipulation, botanical drugs, hypnosis, acupuncture, and other unorthodox therapies. I meet some who understand the importance of placebo responses in good medicine. Most allopaths do not live up to the ideal of their redefined name, however. They remain narrow in their views and quick to condemn the methods of other traditions. They could become allopaths in the better sense of the word by being more open to other approaches to prevention and treatment, especially those drawing on the vast power of the mind. By doing so, they might also gain more respect from a public now drawn in desperation to alternative practitioners.

I would like to see allopaths take a hard look at where their system is leading. What will medical costs be in the year 2000 if present trends continue? What will be the incidence of iatrogenic illness? What will be the effect of the glut of useless scientific information on medical school teaching and the medical literature? Will public health really be better than today or will cancer be striking one in every three or two rather than one in every four, even as methods of treating it improve?

I urge practitioners of all systems of medicine to work more at preventing illness. That will mean learning more about the true causes of disease and teaching people how to recognize and manage its early stages. Education ought to be one of the primary activities of doctors. Mystification may seem a reasonable way to protect the trade secrets of a medical guild, but it is not really in the larger interests of either doctors or patients. There is plenty of mystery about health and illness without adding to it. I hope physicians of the coming century will be able to acknowledge the irreducible mysteries at the core of medical reality while realizing that educating patients about prevention and treatment will make their day-to-day jobs significantly easier.

All of these changes will follow naturally as doctors construct new and better conceptual models of health and healing. Models including consciousness as a determinant of health will open up possibilities for the prevention and management of disease by methods less dangerous, less costly, and more effective than many in favor today.

If researchers and practitioners are slow to meet these challenges and prepare for the twenty-first century, patients should lose no time in getting down to work now. The primary responsibility for health is the patient's. Anyone can learn to keep himself relatively healthy most of the time and to recognize and correct most deviations from health without consulting professional practitioners, whether orthodox or unorthodox. By way of encouragement, let me assure the reader that most of what I know about keeping myself in good health I did not learn in my training as a medical doctor. I learned it from observation of myself and others, from intuition and thought, and from my own experience. You can do the same.

The only prerequisite for learning to take responsibility for one's own health is to discard concepts that stand in the way and adopt more useful ones. It is not just scientists who benefit from new conceptual models. Anyone who comes to see healing as an innate capacity of the body rather than something to be sought outside it will gain greater power over the fluctuations of health and illness. Anyone who recognizes the importance of mind and belief in determining responses to treatments will be able to make better sense of past interactions with medical practitioners and better decisions about future ones.

The theory of health and healing presented here can help

people be more independent and self-reliant in medical matters. It can inspire them to learn their bodies' normal patterns of change, to recognize early signs and symptoms of illness, to experiment with simple methods of treatment, and to be wary of the pitfalls of unthinking confidence in professional doctors. It ought to convince the reader of the potential of the mind to modify physical reality, including diseases of the body and agents that carry them.

The best theory is only an approximation waiting to be replaced by a better one. There are bound to be anomalies left unexplained by this theory of health and healing — bits and pieces of medical reality that do not fit and that I have ignored or tried to sweep under the rug. I am willing to concede the imperfection and incompleteness of this model but think it permits better understanding and control of health and illness than the concepts I infer behind the behavior of most doctors and patients I meet.

Models have a practical purpose: good ones make effective action possible. As the Newtonian model enabled inventors to create the machines of the Industrial Revolution, so this new model of healing can enable all of us to achieve more healthy lives. I have already derived much practical information from it, but I believe changes in thinking must precede changes in action. The ideas in *Health and Healing* are intended to stimulate changes in thinking. I recommend them as good medicine for the intellect. Explanations of disease processes and ways to modify them, techniques of self-diagnosis and self-treatment, ways of taking practical advantage of the interdependence of mind and body — these matters will be the subject of a later book.

NOTES
INDEX

NOTES

2. Like Cures Like, and Less Is More

1. See Trevor M. Cook, *Samuel Hahnemann* (Wellingborough, Northamptonshire, England: Thorsons Publishers, 1981).
2. From a lecture given in 1798 at the University of Pennsylvania, quoted in Martin Kaufman, *Homeopathy in America: The Rise and Fall of a Medical Heresy* (Baltimore: Johns Hopkins University Press, 1971), 3.
3. Kaufman, *Homeopathy in America,* 7–9.
4. Samuel Christian Hahnemann, *Organon of Medicine,* 6th ed. of 1842, translated by William Boericke, M.D. (Calcutta: M. Bhattacharya and Co., Ltd., 1960), 198ff. A new translation (Los Angeles: J. P. Tarcher, 1982) is now available.
5. Cook, *Samuel Hahnemann,* 59.
6. Samuel Christian Hahnemann, *The Chronic Diseases* (New York: 1846), 141–55, quoted in Kaufman, *Homeopathy in America,* 26.
7. Information in the remainder of this chapter comes from Kaufman, *Homeopathy in America,* and from Harris L. Coulter, *Divided Legacy: A History of the Schism in Medical Thought,* vols. 1–3 (Washington, D.C.: Wehawken, 1974–1977).
8. See Richard H. Shryock, *Medicine in America: Historical Essays* (Baltimore: Johns Hopkins University Press, 1966); also the pamphlet *Witches, Midwives, and Nurses: A History of Women Healers* by Barbara Ehrenreich and Deirdre English (Oyster Bay, N.Y.: Glass Mountain Pamphlets, 1972; reprinted in 1973 by Black & Red, Detroit, Mich.).
9. Quoted in Kaufman, *Homeopathy in America,* 87.

3. Why Does Homeopathy Work?

1. Harris L. Coulter, *Homeopathic Science and Modern Medicine: The Physics of Healing with Microdoses* (Richmond, Calif.: North Atlantic Books, 1980), 5.
2. *Journal of the American Institute of Homeopathy* 45 (1952), 162–63.

3. Oliver Wendell Holmes, "Homeopathy and Its Kindred Delusions," two lectures delivered before the Boston Society for the Diffusion of Useful Knowledge, 1842; reprinted in *The Writings of Oliver Wendell Holmes*, vol. 9, *Medical Essays: 1842–1882* (Cambridge, Mass.: The Riverside Press, 1891), 75.

4. Vol. 27 (1957), 563–79.

5. Vol. 44 (1957), 2679–92.

6. Vol. 56, no. 4 (1958), 570–82.

7. K. D. Allanby et al., "Nialamide (Niamid) in Angina Pectoris: Report of a Double-blind Trial," *Lancet*, 21 January 1961, 138–39; F. M. Murphy et al., "Tersavid in Angina Pectoris: A Sequential Clinical Trial," *Lancet*, 21 January 1961, 139–40.

8. R. G. Gibson et al., "Homeopathic Therapy in Rheumatoid Arthritis: Evaluation by Double-blind Clinical Therapeutic Trial," *British Journal of Clinical Pharmacology* 9 (1980), 453–59.

9. Coulter, *Homeopathic Science*, 6, 72.

10. G. Vithoulkas, *The Science of Homeopathy: A Modern Textbook*, vol. 1 (Athens: A.S.O.H.M., 1978), 125.

11. Vol. 23 (1930), 1055–89.

12. Vol. 44 (1954), 6–44.

13. For an analysis of how scientific theory changes, see Thomas Kuhn, *The Structure of Scientific Revolutions* (Chicago: University of Chicago Press, 1962).

4. Health as Wholeness; Wholeness as Perfection

1. John G. Neihardt, *Black Elk Speaks* (Lincoln: University of Nebraska Press, 1961), 35.

2. Ibid., 198–200.

3. Ibid., 198.

4. Isaiah 45:6–7.

5. Lao-tzu, *The Way of Life*, translated by Witter Bynner (New York: Capricorn Books, 1962), 42 (verse 28).

6. See Norman O. Brown, *Hermes the Thief: The Evolution of a Myth* (Madison: University of Wisconsin Press, 1947).

6. Nine Principles of Health and Illness

1. The tendency of the body to maintain equilibrium is called *homeostasis* by physiologists. For a discussion of homeostasis see Walter B. Cannon, *The Wisdom of the Body* (New York: W. W. Norton, 1963; first published in 1932).

2. Lao-tzu, *The Way of Life,* 65–66 (verse 63).
3. See Roger J. Williams, *Biochemical Individuality* (Austin: University of Texas Press, 1956).

7. The Nature of Healing

1. Guido Majno, *The Healing Hand: Man and Wound in the Ancient World* (Cambridge, Mass.: Harvard University Press, 1975), 46–48.
2. Ibid., 105–20.
3. See J. E. Brody, "Fever: New View Stresses Its Healing Benefits," *New York Times,* 28 December 1982, C-1–2; also Matthew J. Kluger, *Fever: Its Biology, Evolution, and Function* (Princeton, N.J.: Princeton University Press, 1979).

8. Allopathic Medicine I: Physicians and Surgeons

1. Ivan Illich, *Medical Nemesis: The Expropriation of Health* (New York: Pantheon, 1976), 2–3.
2. M. H. Roehmer, "Doctor Slowdown: Effects on the Population of Los Angeles County" (Paper presented at session 4054 of the annual meeting of the American Public Health Association, Los Angeles, October 18, 1978).
3. See Oliver Cope, *The Breast: Its Problems — Benign and Malignant — And How to Deal with Them* (Boston: Houghton Mifflin, 1977).
4. E. G. Dimond, C. F. Kittle, and J. E. Crockett, "Comparison of Internal Mammary Artery Ligation and Sham Operation for Angina Pectoris," *American Journal of Cardiology* 5 (1960), 483. For a general evaluation of surgical treatments for coronary artery disease, see Eugene Braunwald, *Heart Disease: A Textbook of Cardiovascular Medicine* (Philadelphia: W. B. Saunders, 1980), 418.
5. L. Rosenthal, "Interview: Denton Cooley — A Change of Heart," *Science Digest,* February 1983, 14.
6. Hippocrates, *Epidemics VI,* chapter 5, translated by W.H.S. Jones and quoted in "From *The Works of Hippocrates*" in *Ways of Health,* edited by David S. Sobel (New York: Harcourt Brace Jovanovich, 1979), 194.
7. R. Dubos, "Hippocrates in Modern Dress," in Sobel (ed.), *Ways of Health,* 205–20.
8. Majno, *The Healing Hand,* 141–206.
9. Stanley Joel Reiser, *Medicine and the Reign of Technology* (Cambridge, Eng.: Cambridge University Press, 1978), 159.

9. Allopathic Medicine II: Materia Medica

1. A. T. Weil, "Botanical vs. Chemical Drugs: Pros and Cons," in *Folk Medicine and Herbal Healing*, ed. George Meyer, Kenneth Blum, and John G. Cull (Springfield, Ill.: Charles C. Thomas, 1981).
2. A. T. Weil, "The Green and the White: Coca and Cocaine," in *The Marriage of the Sun and Moon* by Andrew Weil (Boston: Houghton Mifflin, 1980), 139–65.
3. G. E. Burch, "Experiments of Nature: Whole Leaf and Purified Alkaloids," *American Heart Journal* 83 (1972), 845.
4. *Physicians' Desk Reference* (Oradell, N.J.: Medical Economics Co., published annually).
5. Oliver Wendell Holmes, "Currents and Counter-currents in Medical Science," an address delivered before the Massachusetts Medical Society at its annual meeting, May 30, 1860; reprinted in *The Writings of Oliver Wendell Holmes*, vol. 9, *Medical Essays: 1842–1882* (Cambridge, Mass.: The Riverside Press, 1891), 203.
6. Quoted in Eugene E. Brussell, ed., *Dictionary of Quotable Definitions* (Englewood Cliffs, N.J.: Prentice-Hall, 1970), 150.

10. Allopathic Medicine III: Sins of Omission

1. Lelland Joseph Rather, M.D., quoted in George W. Northrup, *Osteopathic Medicine: An American Reformation* (Chicago: American Osteopathic Association, 1966), 30–31.

11. Some Medical Heresies: Osteopathy, Chiropractic, Naturopathy

1. Northrup, *Osteopathic Medicine*, 3–4.
2. *Autobiography of Andrew Taylor Still, With a History of the Discovery and Development of the Science of Osteopathy* (Kirksville, Mo.: privately published, 1897; a revised edition was published in 1908).
3. Ibid., 31–32.
4. Ibid., 120–22.
5. Ibid., 396–97.
6. Daniel David Palmer, *Text-Book of the Science, Art, and Philosophy of Chiropractic, Founded on Tone* (Portland, Oreg.: Portland Printing House, 1910; reprinted 1966), 18ff.
7. Ibid., 19.
8. Information in this section is taken from Ralph Lee Smith, *At Your Own Risk: The Case Against Chiropractic* (New York: Pocket Books, 1969).

9. See Bartlett Joshua Palmer, *The Bigness of the Fellow Within* (Davenport, Iowa: Chiropractic Fountain Head, 1949); quoted in Smith, *At Your Own Risk.*
10. Quoted in Smith, *At Your Own Risk,* 15.
11. Quoted in Smith, *At Your Own Risk,* 11.
12. Robert Thomson, *The Grosset Encyclopedia of Natural Medicine* (New York: Grosset & Dunlap, 1980), 126–27.
13. Benedict Lust, from an address to the American Naturopathic Association convention of 1925, quoted in his obituary in the *New York Times,* 6 September 1945, 21.
14. René Dubos, *Mirage of Health: Utopias, Progress, and Biological Change* (New York: Harper & Brothers, 1959), 110–11.
15. B. A. Spilker and T. H. Maugh, "How Useful Is Hair Analysis?" *Journal of Energy Medicine* 1:1 (1980), 14.

12. Chinese Medicine

1. See M. Porkert, "Chinese Medicine: A Traditional Healing Science," in Sobel (ed.), *Ways of Health,* 147–72.
2. *The Yellow Emperor's Classic of Internal Medicine (Huang Ti Nei Ching Su Wen),* translated by Ilza Veith, new ed. (Berkeley: University of California Press, 1966), 105.
3. See Ted Kaptchuk, *The Web That Has No Weaver* (New York: Congdon & Weed, 1982).

13. Shamanism, Mind Cures, and Faith Healing

1. For example: Joan Halifax, *Shamanic Voices: A Survey of Visionary Narratives* (New York: E. P. Dutton, 1979); Michael Harner, *The Way of the Shaman: A Guide to Power and Healing* (San Francisco: Harper & Row, 1980).
2. See A. T. Weil, "In the Land of Yagé," in *The Marriage of the Sun and Moon* by Andrew Weil (Boston: Houghton Mifflin, 1980), 99–131; also F. Bruce Lamb, *Wizard of the Upper Amazon: The Story of Manuel Córdova-Rios* (Boston: Houghton Mifflin, 1975).
3. Robert L. Oswalt, *Kashaya Texts, University of California Publications in Linguistics* 36 (1964), 223, 225, 227, 229, 231; quoted in Harner, *The Way of the Shaman,* 128–30.
4. See D. F. Sandner, "Navaho Indian Medicine and Medicine Men," in Sobel (ed.), *Ways of Health,* 117–46.
5. See, for example, Douglas Sharon, *Wizard of the Four Winds: A Shaman's Story* (New York: The Free Press, 1978).

6. Doug Boyd, *Rolling Thunder: A Personal Exploration into the Secret Healing Power of an American Indian Medicine Man* (New York: Random House, 1974).

7. Mary Baker Eddy, *Science and Health with Key to the Scriptures* (Boston: First Church of Christ, Scientist, 1906), 111.

8. Mark Twain (Samuel Clemens), *Christian Science with Notes Containing Corrections to Date* (New York: Gabriel Wells, 1923), 29.

9. *A Century of Christian Science Healing* (Boston: Christian Science Publishing Society, 1966), 65–66.

10. Jerome D. Frank, *Persuasion and Healing: A Comparative Study of Psychotherapy* (Baltimore: Johns Hopkins University Press, 1961), 56.

11. L. D. Weatherhead, *Psychology, Religion, and Healing* (New York: Abingdon-Cokesbury Press, 1951), 153.

12. Frank, *Persuasion and Healing*, 58.

13. H. Rehder, "Wunderheilungen, ein Experiment," *Hippokrates* 26, 577–80, quoted in Frank, *Persuasion and Healing*, 60–61.

14. Psychic Healing

1. See Gary Zukav, *The Dancing Wu Li Masters: An Overview of the New Physics* (New York: Bantam Books, 1980).

2. See Jess Stearn, *Edgar Cayce: The Sleeping Prophet* (New York: Bantam Books, 1968).

3. See John G. Fuller, *Arigo: Surgeon of the Rusty Knife* (New York: Thomas Y. Crowell, 1974).

15. Holistic Medicine

1. See Leslie J. Kaslof, *Wholistic Dimensions in Healing: A Resource Guide* (Garden City, N.Y.: Doubleday, 1978).

2. See David S. Walther, *Applied Kinesiology — The Advanced Approach in Chiropractic* (Pueblo, Colo.: privately published, 1976). The technique is featured in a popular book by John F. Thie with Mary Marks, *Touch for Health* (Santa Monica, Calif.: DeVorss, 1973).

3. See Edward Bach, *Heal Thyself: An Explanation of the Real Cause and Cure of Disease* (London: C. W. Daniel, 1974) and *The Twelve Healers and Other Remedies* (London: C. W. Daniel, 1975).

4. See A. T. Weil, "Reading the Windows of the Soul," in *The Marriage of the Sun and Moon* by Andrew Weil (Boston: Houghton Mifflin, 1980), 181–89.

16. Quackery

1. Stewart H. Holbrook, *The Golden Age of Quackery* (New York: Macmillan, 1959), 123–28.
2. R. Vicker, "How Can You Tell Quack Witch Doctor from Real McCoy?" *Wall Street Journal*, 10 March 1976, 1.
3. Lyman Frank Baum, *The Wizard of Oz* (New York: Bobbs-Merrill, 1900, and many subsequent editions).

19. The Placebo Response

1. *Hooper's Medical Dictionary*, quoted in B. Roueché, "Placebo," in *A Man Named Hoffman and Other Narratives of Medical Detection* by Berton Roueché (Boston: Little, Brown, 1965), 92.
2. O. H. Pepper, "A Note on the Placebo," *American Journal of Pharmacology* 117 (1945), 409–12; cited in R. G. Gallimore and J. L. Turner, "Contemporary Studies of Placebo Phenomena," in *Psychopharmacology in the Practice of Medicine*, edited by Murray E. Jarvik (New York: Appleton-Century-Crofts, 1977), 47.
3. J. S. Goodwin, J. M. Goodwin, and A. V. Vogel, "Knowledge and Uses of Placebos by House Officers and Nurses," *Annals of Internal Medicine* 91 (1979), 106–10.
4. Roueché, *A Man Named Hoffman*, 95.
5. Jerome D. Frank, *Persuasion and Healing: A Comparative Study of Psychotherapy* (Baltimore: Johns Hopkins University Press, 1961), 37.
6. See W. B. Cannon, "Voodoo Death," *Psychosomatic Medicine* 19, (1957), 182–90.
7. A. K. Shapiro et al., "Placebo-induced Side Effects," *Journal of Operational Psychiatry* 6:1 (1974), 43–46.
8. Louis Lasagna, M.D., professor of clinical pharmacology and medicine at Johns Hopkins University School of Medicine, quoted in Roueché, *A Man Named Hoffman*, 110–11.
9. Roueché, *A Man Named Hoffman*, 111.
10. Gallimore and Turner, "Contemporary Studies," 50–52.
11. W. N. Pahnke, "Drugs and Mysticism: An Analysis of the Relationship Between Psychedelic Drugs and the Mystical Consciousness" (Ph.D. diss., Harvard University, 1963).
12. See H. Benson and M. Epstein, "The Placebo Effect: A Neglected Asset in the Care of Patients," *Journal of the American Medical Association* 232:12 (1975), 1225–27; H. Brody, "The Lie That Heals: The Ethics of Giving Placebos," *Annals of Internal Medicine* 97 (1982),

112–18; and Michael Jospe, *The Placebo Effect in Healing* (Lexington, Mass.: Lexington Books, 1978).

20. Medical Treatments as Active Placebos

1. N. E. Zinberg, "Heroin Use in Vietnam and the United States," *Archives of General Psychiatry* 26 (1972), 486–88. L. N. Robins, "A Follow-up of Vietnam Drug Users," Special Action Office Monograph, Series A, no. 1 (Washington, D.C.: U.S. Government Printing Office, 1973). L. N. Robins, D. H. Davis, and D. W. Goodwin, "Drug Use in U.S. Army Enlisted Men in Vietnam: A Follow-up on Their Return Home," *American Journal of Epidemiology* 99 (1974), 235–49. L. N. Robins, J. E. Helzer, M. Hesselbrock, and E. Wish, "Vietnam Veterans Three Years After Vietnam," in *Yearbook of Substance Abuse*, edited by Leon Brill and Charles Winick (New York: Human Sciences Press, 1979).
2. D. Sobel, "Placebo Studies Are Not Just 'All in Your Mind,'" *New York Times*, 6 January 1980, sec. 4, p. 9.
3. J. D. Levine, N. C. Gordon, and H. L. Fields, "The Mechanism of Placebo Analgesia," *Lancet*, 23 September 1978, 654–57; A. Goldstein, "Endorphins and Addiction," in *Classic Contributions in Drug Addiction*, edited by Howard Shaffer and Milton E. Burglass (New York: Brunner-Mazel, 1981), 421–32.
4. A. T. Weil, N. E. Zinberg, and J. M. Nelsen, "Clinical and Psychological Effects of Marijuana in Man," *Science* 162 (13 December 1968), 1234–42.
5. Andrew Weil, *The Natural Mind: A New Way of Looking at Drugs and the Higher Consciousness* (Boston: Houghton Mifflin, 1972); *The Marriage of the Sun and Moon* (Boston: Houghton Mifflin, 1980); and (with Winifred Rosen) *Chocolate to Morphine: Understanding Mind-Active Drugs* (Boston: Houghton Mifflin, 1983).

21. Powers of the Mind and the Problem of Harnessing Them

1. Roy Wallis and Peter Morley (eds.), *Marginal Medicine* (New York: The Free Press, 1976), 27.
2. See Herbert Benson, *The Relaxation Response* (New York: William Morrow, 1975).
3. See Gary E. Schwartz and Jackson Beatty (eds.), *Biofeedback: Theory and Research* (New York: Academic Press, 1977).
4. See, for example, Wilhelm Reich, *The Function of the Orgasm* (New York: Simon & Schuster, 1974).

5. J. Doherty, "Hot Feat: Firewalkers of the World," *Science Digest*, August 1982, 67–71. See also the letter to the editor in response to this article, "Atheist Firewalkers," *Science Digest*, November 1982, 11.

6. Wilder Penfield, *The Mystery of the Mind: A Critical Study of Consciousness and the Human Brain* (Princeton, N.J.: Princeton University Press, 1975).

22. What Doctors Can Learn from Physicists

1. Albert Einstein and Leopold Infeld, *The Evolution of Physics* (New York: Simon & Schuster, 1938), 31.

2. Lord Kelvin (Sir William Thomson), "Nineteenth-century Clouds over the Dynamical Theory of Heat and Light," *Philosophical Magazine* 2 (1901), 1–40.

3. T. Ferris, "Physics' Newest Frontier," *New York Times Magazine*, 26 September 1982, 36.

4. Einstein and Infeld, *Evolution of Physics*, 152.

5. Lincoln Barnett, *The Universe and Dr. Einstein*, 2nd rev. ed. (New York: William Sloane Associates, 1957), 52.

6. See, for example, Fritjof Capra, *The Tao of Physics* (Boulder, Colo.: Shambala Publications, 1975); Gary Zukav, *The Dancing Wu Li Masters: An Overview of the New Physics* (New York: Bantam Books, 1980).

7. See Fred Alan Wolf, *Taking the Quantum Leap: The New Physics for Nonscientists* (San Francisco: Harper & Row, 1981).

8. A rare exception is the book *Space, Time & Medicine* by Larry Dossey (Boulder, Colo.: Shambala Publications, 1982). Dr. Dossey is a clinical physician who perceives the implications of the new physics for his field. See also Harold Bursztajn, Richard L. Feinbloom, Robert M. Hamm, and Archie Brodsky, *Medical Choices, Medical Chances: How Patients, Families, and Physicians Can Cope with Uncertainty* (New York: Delta/Seymour Lawrence, 1983), 1–84.

9. M. M. Cohen, K. Hirshhorn, and W. A. Frosch, "In Vivo and In Vitro Chromosomal Damage Induced by LSD-25," *New England Journal of Medicine* 227 (1967), 1043.

10. See J. H. Tjio, W. N. Pahnke, and A. A. Kurland, "LSD and Chromosomes: A Controlled Experiment," *Journal of the American Medical Association* 210 (1969), 849; and N. I. Dishotsky et al., "LSD and Genetic Damage," *Science* 172, 30 April 1971, 431; also the discussion of the episode in Andrew Weil, *The Natural Mind: A New Way of Looking at Drugs and the Higher Consciousness* (Boston: Houghton Mifflin, 1972), 44–46.

INDEX

abrasions, healing of, 65
"Account of Foxglove and Some of Its Medicinal Uses" (Withering), 102
active placebo, 211–16; medical treatment as, 219–33; psychoactive drugs as model of, 221–26, 232; surgery as, 226; three dimensions of belief, 226–27; brain chemistry and, 227–30; endorphins and, 229–30; practitioners' resistance to use of, 230–31; tetracycline and, 231; marijuana as, 231–32
acupuncture, 96, 143, 147, 148–51, 154–55, 190, 227; theoretical foundation of, 113; and naturopathy, 138; in West, 149–50; for anesthesia, 150–51, 154–55; *see also* Chinese medicine
acute medical emergencies, 82
acute surgical emergencies, 82
acute trauma, 82
adaptation as component of healing, 68, 71–72
adenoids, 86
adrenaline, 242–43
Age of Heroic Medicine, 12–14, 92, 123, 265
agents of disease, 55–56, 120
"Airs, Waters, and Places" (Hippocrates), 91
alcohol, 23, 222, 232, 265
alcoholism, 73
allergies, 83; skin, 19n; and psychoactive drugs, 241–42, 245
allopathic medicine, 8, 8n, 193–95; and Age of Heroic Medicine, 12–

14; definition of, 17, 22, 272; in America, 20, 22–25; in conflict with homeopathy, 22–25; AMA, 22–24; successes of, 24; current criticism of, 25, 81–83; and Law of Infinitesimals, 33–38; and nine principles of health and illness, 52–62; current status of, 81; for acute problems, 82; areas of ineffectiveness, 83; narrow perspective of, 83, 115, 272; medicine vs. surgery, 84–85; merits and demerits of surgery, 84–89; Hippocratic medicine, 90–92; diagnosis in, 92–95; pharmacology, 96–111; drug toxicity, 96–97; sins of omission, 113–22; deficiency in theory and philosophy, 113–16; concentration on disease and illness, 114–16; use of battle and war imagery, 114–15; materialistic bias of, 115; case examples of practical problems resulting from conceptual limitations of, 116–22; and osteopathy, 127–28; and chiropractic, 131; and naturopathy, 137, 138, 139; vs. Chinese medicine, 143, 151, 152, 153–54; and Christian Science, 167–68; and holistic medicine, 181, 183, 184–85, 187–88; and placebo response, 207–18; and science, 257–60, 265–70; denial of significance of consciousness in health, 260; training in, 266; and physics, 267; need for future research, 269–74; need for reform in, 272–74